Longevity Made Easy

Longevity Made Easy

Dr. Damon Cozamanis, D.C.

iUniverse, Inc.
New York Lincoln Shanghai

Longevity Made Easy

iUniverse books may be ordered through booksellers or by contacting:

iUniverse
2021 Pine Lake Road, Suite 100
Lincoln, NE 68512
www.iuniverse.com
1-800-Authors (1-800-288-4677)

This book contains information relating to health care. It is intended as a reference manual only and should not be used as a substitute for any treatment that may have been prescribed by your doctor. It is recommended that you seek your doctor's advice before embarking on the Longevity Made Easy program. All efforts have been made to assure the accuracy of the information presented in this book as of the date of publication. The publisher and the author disclaim liability for any medical outcomes that may occur as a result of applying the methods suggested in this book.

ISBN-13: 978-0-595-41184-9 (pbk)
ISBN-13: 978-0-595-85541-4 (ebk)
ISBN-10: 0-595-41184-3 (pbk)
ISBN-10: 0-595-85541-5 (ebk)

Printed in the United States of America

Contents

Acknowledgements

Seeing this book come to fruition has been one of the great pleasures of my life. There are so many people I have to thank for this book. First and foremost, I would like to thank Dick Walters for his inspiration and the knowledge and principles that he instilled in me at an early age. You left this world way too early. Your spirit still lives on.

I would also like to thank all of the wonderful individuals I have met and trained with over the years who have inspired me to constantly challenge myself and always seek new and smarter ways to achieve my health and fitness goals. Big shout outs go to my brothers Steve and Dion, and my friends and training partners Samson, Nick, and Marcus (5 am workouts rock!).

Additionally, I would like to thank my editor Lorra Garrick. Her insightful editing and thoughtful approach helped to shape this book into what it is today.

Last but not least, I wish to thank Liz for her support, patience and love. You have sacrificed so much for me throughout your life. This book is dedicated to you.

Preface

As a chiropractor and nutritionist in private practice, I regularly hear desperate pleas for help from patients battling an array of ailments. Many of the patients I see on a regular basis are unhealthy due to the poor lifestyle choices they have made. As a result, their bodies have become a breeding ground for illness and disease. There are few people today who actually die of old age. Instead, heart attacks, strokes, cancer, and diabetes are the typical causes of death. If you speak to most people, you'll soon realize that arthritis, digestive disorders, being overweight and lacking energy are a normal part of their lives. As a result, many of them have become dependent on a host of dangerous drugs and surgical procedures just to get through the day.

If you're like most people, you are looking to maintain or improve your health and increase your odds of living a long and healthy life. You wish to reduce your chances of developing illness and disease, staying mentally sharp and remaining physically active as you get older. As you have probably already discovered, there is not shortage of how-to health books on the market, many of which offer counterintuitive and contradictory advice. How do you make sense of everything you hear?

Longevity Made Easy is the result of both a personal and professional quest, one that I am pleased to share with you. This book explains in simple terms how lifestyle changes affect your risk of disease, regardless of whether you have inherited "good" or "bad" genes.

You will quickly learn that it's not as hard as you might think it is to improve your health and to increase your chances of living a long and active life. *Longevity Made Easy* arms you with just the facts presented in a simple and easy to follow format. Whether your goal is to overcome a specific illness or disease, or to maximize your lifespan, *Longevity Made Easy* can help by optimizing your body's natural defense mechanisms. Lets get started...

Introduction

Golden Years? Or Gray Years?

What kind of life would you like to be leading in your "golden" years? That question usually evokes pleasant images of a leisurely retirement, spending time playing with the grandchildren, traveling, and finally pursuing all of the hobbies and interests you never had time for during your working years. Everyone tends to think they'll be chipper and spry well into "old age."

But look around and see what the reality is. Most "old people" are just that: old and wasted away. Rather than having fun out in the sunshine playing catch with a grandchild, many will instead be permanently stuck inside the house, watching through the window from the confinement of a bed or wheelchair.

We've become a very unhealthy, unfit nation, and this is tragically reflected in the appearance of older folks. Senior men have protruding bellies, scrawny legs and slumped posture. Senior women are withered away by brittle bones. Or they're covered in layers of fat. Both genders typically begin each day with a dizzying array of medications. Their calendars are filled with appointments to visit the doctor, not the tennis court. Pain is a part of everyday life. A good day is when they can get up the stairs without any aches. And these are people who are only—yes, I said "only"—70 years old! To a 10-year-old child, that's ancient. But to longevity researchers, that's middle age. Or should be.

Seventy should be young. 110 is old. Unfortunately, it seems that the majority of people just barely into retirement sludge along to cover just 50 yards. They are out of breath and achy from even this mild exertion. Well, that's just part of getting old, right? Wrong! It happens because we let it happen. Of course, nobody thinks they'll end up this way. Somehow, magically, everything will turn out OK. But in reality, it does not work out OK, and almost all people who delude themselves with this way of thinking will end up virtually crippled and chronically ill. Why? Because these people have failed to plan. They waited until they were 69 to start exercising or eating right. That's like waiting until you're 69 to open up an investment fund. Not a smart strategy. The sooner you begin life-extension practices, the longer and healthier you'll live. And maybe when you're 70, you'll be offering to help shovel your 55-year-old neighbor's driveway.

There should be more to life expectancy, however, than just how long a person can breathe. Even a very sick person can live a long life with the most advanced medical care. There's a difference between merely prolonging illness and pain, and actually having more vibrant years to enjoy. That's why it's such a misnomer when we speak of "health" insurance.

Health care is actually "sick care," addressing physical problems after they've already afflicted us. But just think how much better off we'd be if we took preventative measures to avoid getting sick in the first place. Stop believing the lie that all disease and illness is in your genes and there's nothing you can do about it. That's just an excuse to be lazy and live a sedentary, unhealthy lifestyle. Most illness is in fact very preventable if you only follow some common sense rules when it comes to how to treat your body. Far too many people lavish TLC on their houses, cars and other possessions while letting their own bodies fall into disrepair. That simply makes no sense.

Experts are only beginning to understand the various factors that allow some people to live to 100—and with a high quality of life, minus a slow gait—while others drop off much sooner. Living to 100 doesn't have to mean spending the last quarter of your life shriveled in a wheelchair or gasping for each breath in a hospital. Ninety percent of those making it to 100 remain functionally independent into their early 90s. The problem is that very few people make it to 100.

We all know that your chances of reaching a ripe old age in a healthy state are a result of genetics and lifestyle. But how much actually depends on each factor? If your parents passed away at an early age, you're likely to believe that you'll follow suit. Others may have the mindset that, because their parents have lived well into their 90s, that they themselves can live an unhealthy lifestyle without consequence.

If genes are the most telling factor in life expectancy and health, then you'd presume that identical twins would die at about the same age (minus from an injury). In 1998, a group of Swedish researchers studied identical twins that were separated at birth and reared apart.

Amazingly, scientists concluded that only about 20 percent to 30 percent of how long we live is genetically determined. The most important factor is lifestyle. Genetics loads the gun, but lifestyle pulls the trigger!

The dismal news is that it takes willpower and determination on your behalf to make the right choices. Many people who are chronically ill follow sabotaging lifestyle patterns and for the most part, rely on prescription drugs to treat or manage their illnesses.

The U.S. Centers for Disease Control divide the causes of illness into these categories: heredity, 18 percent; environment, 19 percent; medical intervention, 10 percent; and lifestyle, 53 percent. This means that 82 percent of the causes of disease are within your control. See what I mean about the pervasive misconception that it's "all in your genes."

Scientists are fiercely studying why the Japanese islands of Okinawa are home to the largest population of centurions. These individuals have not only managed to maximize their life span, but have also remained active; and look decades younger than their actual age. So what sets these individuals apart?

For one, they tend to get plenty of physical and mental exercise. They chop wood and walk just about everywhere. Their diets tend to be low in unhealthy fats and sodium, and abundant in antioxidant-rich fruits and vegetables. The Okinawans usually eat only to the point of 80 percent satiation. Most Americans have poor control over their eating habits and often gorge themselves at each sitting, or at least continue eating past satiation.

So what happens when Okinawans leave the islands and move elsewhere? As expected, they acquire the diet and lifestyle habits of their adopted country and within a decade, their life spans shorten and their rates of heart disease and cancer soar.

You Can Outlive Your Parents

So why do so many of us seem to die off around the same age our parents did? It could be the way we are raised. Our parents usually bring us up the same way they were brought up. If your parents were raised on fat and calorie-rich foods and led a sedentary lifestyle, chances are good you were too. Because most of us live with our parents for approximately 18 years and then continue to maintain the lifestyle we are accustomed to, it's no wonder our health is so closely tied to that of our parents.

Friendships also have an influence. If you hang out with a group of heavy drinkers whose idea of exercise is eating pizza while watching hours and hours of ball games or playing video games, you are likely to adopt their habits as well.

The key issue, caution scientists who study aging, is that of quality of life. The National Center for Health Statistics has estimated that 15 percent of the average American's life, or about 12 years, is spent in an "unhealthy" state (i.e., impaired by disabilities, injuries and/or disease). Among those reaching age 65, five of their remaining years, on average, will be sickly ones.

Nearly 85 percent of the elderly suffer from one or more diseases or health problems. The most frequently occurring health problems among people over age 65 are:

- Arthritis (48 percent)
- High blood pressure (36 percent)
- Heart disease (32 percent)
- Orthopedic impairments (19 percent)
- Diabetes (11 percent)
- Senile dementia (10 percent)

Studies have found dramatic differences in death rates between individuals who follow simple health habits like those described in this book, and people who do not. Individuals who practiced these healthy habits had much lower mortality (death) rates and were estimated to live nine years longer than those who did not implement any of them. In addition, those adhering to healthy lifestyle habits were only half as likely to have suffered disabilities that kept them from work or limited day-to-day activities.

Top Causes of Death by Disease in Men

- Heart disease
- Cancer
- Stroke
- Respiratory disease
- Diabetes
- Flu and pneumonia
- Kidney disease

Top Causes of Death by Disease in Women

- Heart disease
- Cancer
- Stroke
- Respiratory disease
- Alzheimer's disease
- Diabetes
- Flu and pneumonia

Nobody has to get any of these diseases. The likelihood of developing and dying from one of them can be substantially reduced with simple lifestyle changes. Nearly all are preventable through a nutritious diet, regular exercise, stress reduction and other changes described in this book.

So what makes this book so much different than others dealing with health and longevity? *Longevity Made Easy* deletes the endless confusion regarding what's healthy and what's not. We will sort through the muddle and give you what you really need in a nutshell: **just the facts.**

For example, we all know that exercise is valuable. But how much exercise do we really need a week to create an impressive difference? How hard and how long do we need to exercise each day to be vibrant? And what is the best type of exercise? Does housework count as exercise? Whether you are healthy or currently suffering from a life-threatening condition, this book will help.

The Definition of Health

If you really want to live a long and healthy life, it takes planning and dedication. Health is a process, not an event, and many people never achieve good health because they misunderstand the term. Good health is not just the absence of sickness. That would be like saying that wealth is simply the absence of poverty. Good health means living a healthy lifestyle that includes nutritionally sensible eating and a commitment to exercising and taking care of your body. It doesn't just happen—you have to *make* it happen.

Good health should be your goal from this very moment until your last moment on earth. It's not a goal in the sense that you can ever "reach" it, such as climbing to the top of a mountain. Rather, it is a way of life the benefits of which you will enjoy day in and day out for as long as you live. You are really cheating yourself to live any other way.

Sadly, millions of people pay little or no attention to improving their own health. That's why as a nation our people are in such poor physical condition. It's this neglectful way of thinking that's responsible for the majority of chronically sick people in the U.S. Many illnesses and diseases do not become apparent until there are symptoms. Take heart disease, our nation's top killer of both men and women. It is known as **the silent killer** because most people who have the disease are asymptomatic—free of symptoms. It has been estimated that blockages in the coronary arteries need to affect up to 80-90 percent of the artery before symptoms become apparent.

For many people, the first "symptom" of heart disease is a heart attack. If you're lucky enough to survive your first heart attack, you then enter a cycle of crisis management. This typically involves cardiovascular surgery and drugs for the remainder of your life. Most people who have had a heart attack will admit that they felt fine and had no warning signs. Unfortunately for these people, the disease had been progressing since their teenage years, even though they were unaware of it. Heart disease is years in the making. In fact, I can tell you with 100 percent certainty that as you are reading this book, the arteries leading to your heart and brain have already begun to accumulate plaque and become narrow. You may have even had a recent checkup at the doctor's office that merely involved an exam of your vital signs, your weight and blood pressure, and a quick check of your heart and lungs with a stethoscope.

You were assured that you were in "good" health. Thousands of people who have died of heart attacks and from cancer had so-called "normal" physical exams. It always baffles me when I have patients who smoke or don't exercise inform me that their doctor has told them they are in good health.

Even more disturbing are the countless times I see children enter my office carrying a McDonald's Happy Meal in one hand and a can of soda in the other! It's no wonder the rate of childhood obesity in the U.S. continues to swell. The parents of these children are 100 percent to blame, since children are incapable of driving themselves to a fast-food establishment and purchasing this poison.

Another misconception is that healthy lifestyle habits cancel out unhealthy ones. How many times have you met the smoker who takes vitamins to be healthy? How about the "junk food junkie" who walks a few days a week and proclaims to be leading a "healthy" lifestyle? One desirable habit does not erase an undesirable one. If you smoke, you are unhealthy. Period. If you don't exercise regularly, you are unhealthy. Period. And if you eat a diet high in saturated fat and sugar, you are unhealthy. It's as simple as that.

Living a longer and more healthful life is based on the lifestyle decisions we make today. These decisions include your overall attitude and emotional well-being; how you handle stress; alcohol and tobacco intake; dietary patterns; your exercise regimen; proper rest and your overall nutritional status.

As previously mentioned, experts estimate that genetics accounts for only 20-30 percent of how long we live. The rest is up to you. Sure, there is no guarantee that if you follow a healthy lifestyle pattern you will live a longer and more healthful life. But I think it's safe to say that the odds are heavily in your favor if you do.

Follow an unhealthy lifestyle and it's almost certain that you will die sooner than you have been genetically programmed to live. If you are lucky enough to dodge an early death, the quality of your remaining years may make you think you were better off dead. It's no picnic having to depend on other people to get in and out of a car.

The Health Continuum

Health is a dynamic state, meaning that it is always changing depending on the decisions that we make. I prefer to view health as a continuum, with one end representing an optimal state of health and the other end representing death. At various times in our life we may find ourselves at different ends of this spectrum due to our nutritional and lifestyle habits. If we choose to engage in destructive lifestyle habits such as smoking or excess consumption of unhealthy foods, we would shift more towards the premature death side versus the optimal health/longevity side of the continuum.

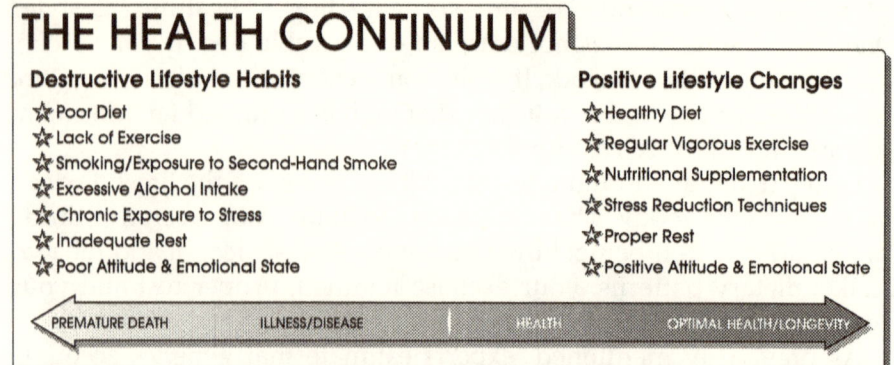

If we continue to engage in such destructive behaviors, our odds of a premature death are increased significantly. If we choose to practice lifestyle habits that promote better health, such as a nutrient-dense diet and sticking to an exercise regimen, we would shift more towards the optimal health end of the continuum and improve our chances of longevity.

The recommendations and guidelines in this book will help ensure that your body is gravitating more towards the optimal health end of the continuum. My longevity plan is based on solid research as well as the personal experiences of many "super seniors" I have interviewed along the way.

These seemingly ageless seniors implemented positive lifestyle changes later in life and now appear far younger physically and mentally than their same-age counterparts. They prove that getting old doesn't have to mean spending your golden years popping pills, seeing doctors, remaining sedentary or relying on a motorized scooter to get around. It is my hope that this book will help inspire you to make rewarding changes in your life and help you realize that it's never too late to start living a vibrant, energetic life.

My longevity plan addresses all aspects of health and will give you the potential to add 10 or more years (not ill years) to your life. **So think about it.** Are you willing to make a few sacrifices today in order to have a much better life tomorrow? If so, make yourself a commitment to stick with the recommendations outlined in this book. These are not temporary changes. They must be adhered to for a lifetime.

Benefits of my *Longevity Made Easy* plan include:

- Increased life span of 10 or more years
- Reduced risk of heart disease, cancer, stroke, diabetes and Alzheimer's disease
- Reduced risk of disability and dependency on others later in life
- Reduced body fat and improved muscle tone
- Increased energy levels
- Improved cognitive function and ability to concentrate
- Improved mood
- Improved self-esteem
- Prevent premature aging and regain a more youthful appearance

I do not recommend just flipping through the pages and picking and choosing which sections you are interested in. They are all equally as important and would not have been included if they did not have a significant impact on health and longevity.

First and foremost, you must be prepared mentally and physically to adopt and incorporate these changes into your life forever, and not just for a few weeks or months. Doing so will only be a waste of your time. Remember, the body that you have right now is the only body that you will ever have during your lifetime, so treat it well and learn how to healthily enjoy all that life has to offer.

Chapter 1

How Long Will YOU Live?

Most people don't take steps to ensure good health until it's too late, usually after they have had a massive heart attack, stroke or are diagnosed with diabetes. Check out your local health club to witness this phenomenon. You will see "old" people shuffling from one machine to the next, not quite sure what they are doing. In fact, some don't have the slightest clue how to perform basic muscle-resistance exercises, and typically use the apparatus incorrectly. In other words, the concept of working out is totally foreign to them. And they are now paying the price.

You just know that they haven't been exercising much in their life, and they've finally come to their senses. All along, they thought they'd been getting exercise with the housework or on the job. But chores and workplace tasks can never replace the type of exercise that promotes bone density, efficient heart-lung capacity and proper spinal alignment. Once you let the combination of old age and lack of structured exercise/proper diet turn what was once a limber stride into a stiff gait, it's often too late to regain most of that lost joint and bone power.

Moreover, even after catastrophic health events, many people continue to live the hazardous lifestyle that jeopardized them in the first place. We've all heard about the person who turns off his oxygen tank to drag on a cigarette.

I've often wondered why some people care so little about their health. They are under the false assumption that a few vitamins each day will keep them strong and kicking, or that some medication will fix any problems that may arise from a toxic lifestyle. The human body is not a car. You just can't get something wrong fixed. The only way to ensure first-rate health is by taking the necessary steps to prevent illness and disease.

I believe the major challenges to improved health and longevity for most people are lack of motivation and determination, and inconvenience. Little baggies of sugary cookies and microwavable foods in boxes are convenient. Vegetables often require rinsing, chopping and careful cooking; and other healthy foods typically require preparation, while fast food, processed foods and single-serving snack cakes need little to none. Exercise requires drive and grit. Drugs and nutritional supplements aimed at weight loss take none. Given these realities, too many people are inclined to take the path of least resistance.

Many people view risky surgical procedures as a way to attain an ideal body weight. Gastric bypass surgery, which drastically shrinks the volume of food that the stomach can hold, is a multi-billion dollar per year industry! Whatever happened to a good old-fashioned 60-minute walk at one's top speed? I'll tell you what happened to it. The TV and a giant bag of tortilla chips and half a liter of soda have replaced it.

So what's the answer? Having someone cut into your stomach to alter nature's design, so that you can no longer cram the entire bag of chips into your gut? This is about as unnatural as solutions come. Gastric bypass surgery is not without the risk of serious—sometimes life-threatening—complications. Furthermore, surgically induced weight loss fails to address the root emotional causes of compulsive overeating.

My *Longevity Made Easy* program gives you the best chance at optimal health and increased life span by targeting the conditions that are most likely to make you ill and lead to an early funeral. And the targeting is done without dangerous drugs and surgery, calorie or point tracking, meetings or food journals.

The overall top 10 causes of death for U.S. men and women combined are:

- Heart disease
- Cancer
- Medical errors (yes, you read that right)
- Stroke
- Chronic lower respiratory ailments
- Accidents
- Diabetes
- Alzheimer's disease

- Kidney disease
- Septicemia (infection)

Nearly all of these ailments are linked in one way or another to unhealthy daily patterns such as poor diet, sedentary lifestyle, excess weight and smoking. But actually, that's great news for you! It means that you have the power to change your destiny. The power comes from the area in your brain responsible for decision-making!

The causes of medical errors are many and varied, and include mishaps stemming from surgery, medication administration and hospital-related infections. Of course, the best way to avoid dying from a medical error is to remain healthy, thereby limiting your chances of having to see a doctor or needing to be hospitalized in the first place.

Below, I have outlined the risk factors for some of the more common diseases. If you have one or more risk factors, take immediate action to reduce your risk of developing these deadly conditions, including implementing healthy lifestyle standards and regular screening procedures as outlined in Chapter 9. It's never too late to make a difference.

Heart Disease

"Heart disease" refers to a group of disorders that affect the heart and cardiovascular system. Ninety percent of all heart attacks are related to lifestyle. Therefore, you have a great deal of control—even when heart attacks "run" in your family—when it comes to preventing heart disease.

Controllable Risk Factors

- **Unhealthy diet.** Eating habits based on foods that are processed, fried, sugared up, from animals, full of additives and high-sodium. "Eat everything in moderation" is a very subjective mantra. To some people, "moderation" is four servings a day of an animal-based food such as beef, bacon and fattening cheese.

- **Smoking.** Tobacco smoke damages blood vessels.

- **High blood pressure.** Over time, elevated blood pressure (140/90 or higher) can damage coronary arteries by hardening them. Do whatever it takes to maintain a healthy blood pressure.

- **Elevated LDL ("bad") cholesterol.** The lower your LDL cholesterol is, the lower your risk. In fact, it's a better gauge of risk than total blood cholesterol. LDL cholesterol levels above 130 mg/dL put you at an increased risk for heart attack. Ideally, try to reduce your LDL cholesterol level to 100 mg/dL or lower.

- **Low HDL ("good") cholesterol.** Low levels of HDL cholesterol (< 40 mg/dL) can put you at high risk for heart disease. Your HDL level should be at or above 60 mg/dL.

- **Diabetes.** Risk of heart disease is even higher if your blood sugar (glucose) level isn't well controlled.

- **Obesity.** Excess weight increases the strain on your heart, raises blood pressure, increases cholesterol and bumps up diabetes risk. Also, being overweight tends to discourage people from working up a good sweat. You can't be "healthy and fat."

- **Physical inactivity.** All reputable medical organizations and establishments recognize this as a *major* risk factor for heart disease.

- **Emotions and anger.** These may make you engage in other risk factors, such as battling boredom with cookies and ice cream. Chronic exposure to stress has also been shown to double heart attack risk.

- **Excessive alcohol consumption.** This can raise blood pressure and triglyceride levels.

Uncontrollable Risk Factors

- **Gender.** Men are generally at greater risk than are women for heart disease. However, the risk for women increases after menopause.

- **Heredity and race.** If your siblings, parents or grandparents have heart disease, you are at increased individual risk. Blacks have a higher risk of heart disease and high blood pressure than do Whites. Latinos, American Indians and Native Hawaiians also have an increased risk.

- **Age.** Most people who die of heart disease are over 65. However, with the rising rates of obesity in America, a growing number of younger people are developing early signs of heart disease.

Cancer

Many types of cancer are gender specific or related to harmful lifestyle habits. When it comes to cancer, prevention and early detection are your best options. Many cancers are curable if caught early enough.

Controllable Risk Factors

- **Tobacco exposure.** This reckless yet pervasive habit accounts for one-third of U.S. cancer deaths every year. Even second-hand smoke, which contains about 60 carcinogens, increases lung cancer risk for nonsmokers. The Environmental Protection Agency has classified tobacco smoke as a Class A carcinogen—a known cause of human cancer, and not just of the lungs; it also causes cancer of the bladder, mouth, pancreas, pharynx, larynx, kidney, stomach and esophagus.

- **High-fat diet (bad fats).** A person can be thin and still have a fattening, cancer-inviting diet.

- **Prolonged exposure to UV radiation.** The sun's rays damage DNA and can cause mutations that lead to skin cancer, which can then spread to the lungs and brain. Tanning beds also increase skin cancer risk. People with dark skin are not immune to skin cancer! In fact, repeated *tanning* heightens risk. So if you "never burn," don't assume you can't get skin tumors.

■   **Excessive alcohol intake.** This has been linked particularly to higher breast cancer risk.

■   **Prolonged exposure to radiation or cancer-causing chemicals and toxins.** Repeated exposure to X-rays can be harmful. Speak to your doctor about the need for each X-ray. Repeated exposure to certain chemicals, metals or pesticides can also increase cancer risk.

■   **Hormone replacement therapy (HRT).** Studies have shown that the use of estrogen increases the risk of uterine and breast cancer. Many doctors are now prescribing HRT that includes progesterone along with low doses of estrogen. Progesterone helps counteract estrogen's harmful effect on the uterus. There are still risks; studies have revealed an increase of breast cancer in women who have used estrogen and progesterone together.

■   **Obesity and physical inactivity.** A recent report published in the *New England Journal of Medicine* (2003) estimates that, in the United States, 14 percent of deaths from cancer in men and 20 percent of deaths in women were due to overweight and obesity.

Uncontrollable Risk Factors

■   **Age.** Cancer cells do not "age" like normal cells do. This is why they just grow and grow, invading healthy body tissue, and they are exceptionally skilled at invasion of healthy but aging tissue. Also, an aged body's weak immune system is no match for cancer.

■   **Gender.** Certain cancers are gender-specific such as prostate in men and uterine/breast/ovarian in women.

■   **Race.** Population studies have revealed an associative link between certain cancers and certain races. But some experts believe the higher rate of, for instance, prostate cancer among Black men might be explained by differences in red meat consumption among Blacks, when compared to Whites. An "uncontrollable" risk factor that's tied to race would have to be genetic in origin. To date, no genetic markers specific to race have been identified that increase cancer risk or mortality.

- **Heredity.** A study published in the July 13, 1999, issue of the *Journal of the National Cancer Institute* suggests that weak genes can increase susceptibility to certain cancers. How many of us have heard of that man who smoked two packs of cigarettes a day and made it to 98, while another who smoked only on occasion developed lung cancer and died at 53? We do not have a crystal ball that can tell us how long we'll live, but we can logically assume that exposure to hazardous lifestyle habits and environmental toxins will put us at higher individual risk for cancer.

Stroke

About 700,000 Americans every year are stricken by stroke. A stroke occurs when the blood supply to part of the brain is suddenly interrupted or when a blood vessel in the brain ruptures. Thus, brain cells no longer receive oxygen and nutrients from the blood, and begin to die.

The symptoms of a stroke include the sudden onset of: numbness or weakness, especially on one side of the body; confusion or trouble speaking or understanding speech; trouble seeing in one or both eyes; difficulty walking; dizziness, or loss of balance or coordination; or sudden severe headache with no known origin. Stroke may cause problems with thinking, awareness, attention, learning, judgment and memory. About 25 percent of people who recover from their first stroke will have another stroke within five years.

Controllable Risk Factors

- **High blood pressure.** This is the single most important risk factor for stroke. High blood pressure yields no symptoms, which is why many people have no clue that they have it.

- **Smoking.** This deadly habit is a major, preventable risk factor for stroke. Smoke damages the walls of blood vessels. Smokers who use certain types of birth control pills are at an even greater risk for stroke, especially over age 35.

■ **Diabetes.** While diabetes is treatable, it still increases stroke risk.

■ **High cholesterol.** Because elevated cholesterol is a major risk factor for heart disease, this amplifies stroke risk. Low levels of HDL cholesterol also may raise stroke risk.

■ **Physical inactivity and obesity.** A wealth of research points to these as major risk factors for stroke.

■ **Excessive alcohol intake.** Excessive alcohol intake can lead to high blood pressure and increase the risk for stroke.

Uncontrollable Risk Factors

■ **Heredity and race.** Risk is greater if a parent, grandparent or sibling has had a stroke. Blacks are also more likely to die from a stroke due in part to a higher risk of high blood pressure, diabetes and obesity—but keep in mind that socioeconomic factors are believed to play a role in mortality rates among different races.

■ **Age.** People of all ages, including children, have strokes. But the older you are, the greater your risk.

■ **Gender.** Men in general have a higher risk of stroke than women.

■ **Prior stroke or heart attack.** Having a prior stroke or heart attack increases the risk for a second stroke.

Diabetes

With diabetes, the body does not produce or properly use insulin. Insulin is a hormone that is needed to convert sugar, starches and other food into energy needed for daily life. About 18.2 million people in the U.S. have diabetes; and about 5.2 million are unaware they have it.

Type 1 diabetes results from the body's failure to produce insulin. Type 2 diabetes (90 percent of diagnosed diabetics) results from insulin resistance (a condition in which the body fails to properly use insulin), combined with relative insulin deficiency.

Often, Type 2 diabetes can be "controlled" through radical changes in diet, and exercise. Some Type 2 diabetics take medication. Type 1 diabetics must take insulin injections daily. Experts have not identified any lifestyle choices that raise risk for Type 1 diabetes.

However, being overweight and inactive are profound controllable risk factors for Type 2 diabetes. In fact, strong evidence is clearly exhibited in all the young kids today who are being diagnosed with Type 2 diabetes. What's going on with children today, that was absent several generations ago? Two things: obesity and inactivity.

Controllable Risk Factors

- **Weight and body mass index (BMI).** Excess fat that is stored around the abdomen is more of a health risk than is fat stored in the hips and thighs. A BMI of 20-25 indicates a healthy weight range. If you have a BMI of 25 or more and are not an athlete, you are considered overweight. About 80 percent of Type 2 diabetics are overweight.

- **Impaired glucose tolerance (IGT).** IGT occurs when the blood glucose level is higher than normal, but not high enough to be classified as diabetes. Sometimes referred to as pre-diabetes, one-third of people with IGT will develop diabetes, unless lifestyle changes are made.

- **Abnormal blood lipids.** Having abnormal blood lipid levels, such as HDL cholesterol less than 35 mg/dL, or triglycerides greater than 250 mg/dL, is associated with increased risk.

Uncontrollable Risk Factors

- **Age.** This is an indirect risk factor because older people tend to become less active and gain weight.

- **Family history.** Having a parent or sibling with diabetes. Heredity is the most important predisposing factor for diabetes, especially for Type 1.

- **Gestational diabetes.** Having diabetes during pregnancy, or delivering a baby weighing more than 9 lbs, increases risk.

- **Ethnicity.** People of Black, Latino, Asian and Pacific Islander heritage have a heightened risk.

COPD (Chronic Obstructive Pulmonary Disease)

Ever see someone pulling a small oxygen tank around? Sometimes, the tank is small enough to be wedged in a large purse or waist pack. Tubes run up the person's nose. Usually, these people have some form of chronic obstructive pulmonary disease (COPD).

COPD is a lung disease that's usually caused by smoking. It's estimated that 80-90 percent of all cases of COPD are a direct result of smoking. That overweight, slumped-over, haggard-looking, wrinkled person with the oxygen tank may have very well once been a thin, tall, glowing 25-year-old who thought it was cool to smoke.

COPD includes chronic bronchitis and emphysema. Symptoms of the disorder include shortness of breath, increased mucus and coughing. People with COPD often say it feels like they are trying to breathe through a straw and that they are gasping for air with each breath. Most people fear cancer the most, but emphysema is a terminal condition.

Controllable Risk Factors

- **Smoking.** Even people chronically exposed to secondhand smoke have an increased risk. Some, not all, of the damage caused by smoking is irreversible.

- **Exposure to occupational and environmental pollutants.** This includes dust, ozone, and gases or chemicals such as traffic exhaust fumes.

- **Periodontal disease.** People with periodontal disease have one and a half times the risk for developing COPD than those without periodontal disease. It is believed that the bacteria responsible for periodontal problems can travel into the lungs and cause inflammation and infection.

Uncontrollable Risk Factors

- **Age.** This is partly related to the number of years of smoking.

- **Gender.** COPD is much more common in men than in women, but this may be largely related to the higher rate of smoking among men.

- **Ethnic background.** COPD is more common in Whites, despite high rates of smoking among Blacks and other racial and ethnic groups.

- **Medical conditions.** A history of frequent childhood lung infections.

Alzheimer's Disease

Alzheimer's Disease (AD) is named after Dr. Alois Alzheimer, a German doctor. In 1906, Dr. Alzheimer noticed changes in the brain tissue of a woman who had died of an unusual mental illness. He found abnormal plaques and tangled bundles of nerve fibers in her brain during an autopsy. These plaques and tangles in the brain are considered signs of AD.

It has been estimated that as many as 4.5 million Americans suffer from AD. The disease usually begins after age 60, and risk continues to increase with age. Over time, AD causes severe short-term memory loss and incoherent thinking. Eventually, victims of this incurable illness fail to recognize family members, and die from physical complications of the disease.

It is important to note that AD is not a normal part of aging. The risk for AD can be reduced considerably through modification of specific controllable risk factors listed below. Many of these are still under investigation.

Controllable Risk Factors

- **Lack of intellectual and physical activity.** When the mind is stimulated through intellectual pursuits, the size and structure of neurons and the connections between them actually change. Research presented at the Proceedings of the National

Academy of Sciences (2002) suggests that people who engage in *fewer* physical, leisure and intellectual activities are almost four times more likely to develop Alzheimer's than those who remain active, both physically and mentally. Reading books and newspapers; playing cards or board games such as backgammon, checkers or chess; or playing a musical instrument were correlated with a lower risk. Also, the more frequent the activity, the lower the risk. People who do crossword puzzles four days a week have been shown to have almost half the risk of those who do them once a week, according to a recent study appearing in the *New England Journal of Medicine* (2003). Just how brain exercise may influence AD risk has not been established scientifically.

■ **Elevated homocysteine levels in the blood.** Research published in the journals *Stroke* and the *New England Journal of Medicine* showed that persons with elevated homocysteine are two to three times more likely to develop AD than those with normal levels.

■ **High blood pressure or high cholesterol.** People with high blood pressure or high cholesterol levels in midlife are twice as likely to develop AD in later life than are people with normal blood pressure and cholesterol levels, according to a study published in the *British Medical Journal* (2001). High blood pressure and high cholesterol are thought to increase the risk of AD by inducing atherosclerosis (hardening of the arteries), and thus impairing blood flow to the brain.

■ **Cardiovascular disease.** People with cardiovascular disease have been found to have a 30 percent higher risk of developing dementia, including both AD and vascular dementia, according to a study presented at the 2002 annual meeting of the American Geriatric Society. The results of this study and others with similar findings suggest that prevention of cardiovascular disease may be the most effective deterrent we have for dementia.

■ **Stroke.** A stroke needn't be severe to increase risk of Alzheimer's. Strokes often occur without symptoms, and the damage they leave behind is detectable only by an MRI scan. A study of over 1,000 older persons as part of the Rotterdam Scan Study found that people with MRI evidence of silent strokes were more than twice as likely during a 3.5-year period to develop dementia than those without such brain damage. Obesity, high blood pressure and high cholesterol levels at midlife each doubled the risk of dementia later in life, says a study reported in the *Archives of Neurology* (2003). It is thought that each of these conditions cause damage to the delicate arteries that supply the brain with oxygen and nutrients.

■ **History of brain trauma.** This means damage from disease that affects the circulatory system, like high blood pressure and physical trauma to the head and brain.

Uncontrollable Risk Factors

■ **Age.** The likelihood of developing Alzheimer's approximately doubles every five years after age 65. About 5 percent of men and women 65-74 have AD, and nearly half of those over 85 may have the disease.

■ **Family history and genetics.** People who have a parent or sibling with Alzheimer's are two to three times more likely to develop it than those who do not. The more people in your family who have the illness, the greater your risk. Scientists have also identified specific genes that are associated with an individual's risk of AD, but this does not guarantee that the individual will develop it.

Some Important Points

No family history of a particular disease in no way means you are at low risk, or that you can be careless with eating or exercise habits. Think of it this way: If you didn't inherit your mother's short stature, father's hair color, grandmother's tendency to freckle, and grandfather's big ears, what makes you think you inherited their "longevity genes?"

Secondly, one might wonder why an animal-based diet can be unhealthy, since humans evolved on meat in the first place. Early man hunted beasts and feasted on their muscle. However, because they actually had to hunt for their meat as opposed to stopping at a drive-through or picking it up at the supermarket, they ate meat only when there was a kill, which in some cases may have taken weeks. Moreover, this meat was wild, and therefore a lot leaner and healthier than the meats we consume today.

Early man also supplemented this meat-based diet with plenty of berries, fruits and vegetables, picked fresh and pure without pesticides. His animal-based diet excluded processed, sugary foods! Furthermore, early man was very physically active.

Today's meat-based diet is accompanied by an assault of junky snack foods, sodas and extreme inactivity, not to mention all sorts of environmental toxins.

In a Nutshell

As you can see, nearly every one of the top causes of death by disease in the U.S. are linked in one way or another to unhealthy daily patterns such as poor diet, sedentary lifestyle, excess weight and smoking. The good news is that you do not have to become another statistic and can delay or prevent these top killers by adhering to the lifestyle recommendations outlined in this book. Implementing and adhering to these recommendations will give you the best shot at maximizing the number of years you live and the quality of those years. As you will soon learn, it is possible to increase your life expectancy by 10 or more years no matter how genetically-challenged you may be (or think you may be).

Chapter 2

Change Your Mind—Change Your Health

Life Extension Value: 8–10 Years

"Our attitude towards life determines life's attitude toward us."
John C. Maxwell

Consider for a moment the last time you had a truly great day. Perhaps you awakened feeling rested and energized, ready to embrace the world. As the day progressed, you felt more confident and happy. Small, pleasant events began to accumulate. Perhaps you found a forgotten five-dollar bill in your pants pocket, received a letter from an old friend, got an unexpected refund, closed a deal, and actually enjoyed your day at the office. It all began with those first thoughts in your head, "I feel great!" You began the day with a refreshing state of mind and a positive attitude.

Now contrast that experience with the last bad day you had. You didn't even want to get out of bed. You considered calling in to work sick and sleeping all day huddled beneath the covers. You dreaded the hours ahead. Maybe you cut yourself shaving, locked the keys in the car, left your lunch at home, or forgot a big meeting. Your day never got any better from the first moment you told yourself, "This day's gonna be lousy!" You were the same person on both days, but your thoughts, feelings and emotions differed dramatically. Not surprisingly, so did the outcomes.

One of the most powerful prescriptions for a healthy body can't be stuffed in a capsule or elixir at the health food store. Every person uses it daily. It's affordable and comes from a completely renewable source—so it's always available to those who want it. It has been the subject of medical research for many years: A healthy body begins with a healthy mind. The power of your mind can be harnessed to improve your health and help you live beyond expectancy.

We all spend much of our day in dialogue with ourselves. In most situations we hear a voice in our heads that is amplifying our thoughts. These thoughts, and our subsequent attitudes about our circumstances, influence our overall health.

Mind Over Matter

Imagine that you've been experiencing pain for several weeks, which has just been diagnosed as cancer. You enroll in an experimental drug study. Although the drug has not yet been approved for use on those afflicted with cancer, you are hopeful that it will provide the cure. During the trial, you begin to feel dramatically better. The doctors tell you that your cancer has gone into remission. As you prepare to praise the medical treatment, you learn that your progress is the result of a sugar pill: a placebo.

Well, not exactly the sugar pill. You actually owe your progress to faith, your faith in the treatment that you were receiving. You could have gotten the same results with the same level of faith in a doorknob. This "placebo effect" has been documented since the 1950s, but until recently the medical community dismissed it as merely a feat of self-deception. Now, however, researchers are learning that our expectations can profoundly affect the outcome of illness and disease.

The placebo effect has been one of the most constant indications that a wide variety of conditions can be positively affected by an as-yet unknown internal system in virtually every person. Among those conditions that have proven responsive to placebo treatment are angina pectoris, cancer, rheumatoid arthritis, warts, asthma, ulcers, migraine headaches, allergies, multiple sclerosis, diabetes and psychiatric disorders.

While modern medicine focuses on treating the body, it's the mind and its work that hold the amazing power to positively impact our healthiness. Documented cases exist of people whose cancer spontaneously went into remission. Such patients had a common link: Before the remission, they developed a more upbeat attitude toward their illness.

Even though few people leave their doctors' offices with a prescription for a positive mental attitude, ample scientific and medical evidence prove the importance of our thoughts, emotions and outlooks toward our overall physical stability. Consider these examples:

- The American Psychological Association's *Journal of Personality and Social Psychology* reports: "A positive mental attitude can add more years to your life than exercise and is more important than other known influences on survival, such as loneliness, gender, body weight, tobacco use, blood pressure and cholesterol."

- Results of a 15-year study of aging and Alzheimer's disease in nuns suggest that a positive emotional state at an early age may help ward off illness and disease and prolong life. Researchers found that the nuns who articulated more positive emotions in their autobiographies lived as much as 10 years longer than those expressing fewer upbeat emotions.

- A Dutch study found that people who described themselves as being highly optimistic had lower rates of cardiovascular death and a lower risk of death from all causes than people who said they were highly pessimistic. Those who reported considerable levels of optimism had a 55 percent lower risk of death from all causes and a 23 percent lower risk of cardiovascular death than people who reported elevated levels of doomful expectations of life.

On average, optimists can expect to live almost 20 percent longer than pessimists. These findings arose from a study published in the *Mayo Clinic Proceedings*. People with encouraging attitudes not only suffer from fewer and less severe diseases than those with negative outlooks, but actually live much lengthier and robust lives. Researchers estimate that having a positive forecast can augment your life expectancy by an average of 8 years.

A positive approach does not pop into your mind by itself. How you feel is a decision you must make every day. These findings tell us what many have known all along—the mind and body are in fact linked, and our attitude has an impact on the final outcome: death.

Negative Thoughts and Emotions Damage the Body

Research clearly indicates that a positive mental attitude impacts health and longevity, but how do negative thoughts and emotions contribute to poor health and a reduced life expectancy? Researchers are not sure at this time, but many believe that negative emotional states such as anger, hatred, grief, depression, and anxiety have a cumulative effect on the body over time. They believe that these downbeat emotional conditions adversely affect the immune system and significantly increase a person's risk for disease, handicap and death. Keep in mind that it's the immune system that protects our bodies against foreign invaders that have the potential to make us sick. When this system functions sub-optimally, the likelihood of illness increases significantly.

Research continues to demonstrate links between our state of mind and the health of our immune system. A relatively new area of study, called psychoneuroimmunology, or PNI, has emerged from this scientific interest in the connection between the brain, the nervous system and the immune system. PNI attempts to unveil the complex connection between the mind and body and determine to what extent psychological state influences health. PNI studies have revealed strong scientific evidence to suggest that psychological factors such as stress, depression and grief influence the onset of physical decline.

Your brain has the ability to communicate with your body, and vice versa, with the help of nerves, neurons and special chemical messengers known as neurotransmitters. Together, these structures allow the brain to send signals to all tissues in the body and influence their behavior. Chemicals released by the brain also have the ability to affect the behavior of the immune system. This, in turn, can increase or decrease your resistance to sickness. Nerves leaving the brain activate numerous other structures, such as muscles, internal organs, and even the walls of arteries and veins to further influence the functioning of our bodies. The entire body is literally "wired" by the brain.

That school-test-day ailment was all in your head, and the extensive network led by your brain coordinated the whole affair. When we recognize this connection between the nervous system and the immune system, it's not surprising that certain psychological states affect our body's ability to ward off disorders.

Numerous studies in the field of PNI suggest that people can voluntarily enhance their immune systems by changing their thoughts, emotions and attitudes to a more positive state. In rare instances, this has led to near-miraculous results, something the medical profession refers to as "spontaneous remission."

Over the past 20 years, mind-body medicine has provided considerable evidence that psychological factors can play a substantive role in the development and progression of coronary artery disease, the number one cause of death in the United States. There is also considerable evidence that emotional traits, both negative and positive, influence people's susceptibility to infection. Individuals who report higher levels of stress or negative moods have been shown to develop more severe illness than those who report less stress or more positive moods.

Studies at Yale and Rutgers Universities by Ellen Idler, Ph.D., Professor of Sociology at Rutgers, and Stanislav Kasl, Ph.D., Professor of Epidemiology at Yale, revealed that the opinion of one's health status—how well one thinks one is—may be the best predictor of well-being and future health.

However, this doesn't mean that a person could neutralize the harmful effects of bad diet and lack of exercise by convincing himself that he's as healthy as a horse. In fact, there exist plenty of people who believe they're in "great shape," even though they don't exercise and eat too much of the wrong foods or ingredients. There's no such thing as being in great shape in the absence of consistent cardio and strength-training workouts, no matter what one thinks.

Attitude will not make bones denser or joints stronger. Positive thinking will not make the heart pump more blood with each beat, or strengthen muscle fibers. But if you feel good about yourself, you are more likely to stick to an exercise regimen and feed your body healthy foods, than if you feel crummy about yourself!

That should be a wake-up call for people of all ages: Start believing that you are fit and strong and that you will live a long and healthy life. This belief, in and of itself, will not extend the life span of your body's cells and heart muscle. But it will get you pumped up enough to be more excited about life, and this thrill will inspire you to make smarter food choices and commit yourself to exercise.

A Healthy State of Mind

It may be premature to conclude that a positive attitude and positive thoughts and emotions are the keys to good health, but we cannot discount the fact that implementing these changes enhances the effectiveness of the body's defenses and healing mechanisms, potentially improving our states of health. By becoming actively involved in self-healing, one shifts from feelings of helplessness and hopelessness to those of control and optimism. And, as we have seen, optimism leads to a longer life.

An impressive list of ailments has been successfully treated with techniques that utilize the mind as a tool for healing the body, demonstrating just how powerful the mind/body connection can be. Just as these illnesses and conditions can be treated using the mind, some can also be caused by wayward thoughts and emotions.

- Tension headaches
- Chronic fatigue syndrome
- Insomnia
- Depression
- Neck and low back pain
- Muscle spasms and tension
- High blood pressure
- Cardiovascular disease
- Colitis and other bowel inflammations
- Irritable bowel syndrome
- Stomach ulcers
- Premenstrual syndrome
- Infertility
- Chronic pain syndrome
- Certain forms of cancer
- HIV/AIDS

Unfortunately, even with evidence of the powerful mind/body connection, the medical community still encourages the division of mind and body by often ignoring the mind and treating only physical symptoms. Many doctors today view the body as merely parts and organs, rather than as components of a complex and integrated system that rely upon the proper functioning of the others to perform their duties satisfactorily, undermining the reality that every part of the body affects each other in some way. These physicians commonly sell their patients on the idea that health is simply the absence of disease. That's similar to believing that wealth is the absence of poverty, or that sunshine is the absence of rain.

This is a major problem with conventional medicine in general. Most doctors during a routine physical exam will ask the patient a few questions, check their vital signs, palpate and percuss specific areas of a patient's body and perform a brief visual inspection, then proclaim the patient to be in excellent health. This only motivates the patient to continue living his or her current lifestyle, which may include little to no exercise, a diet excessive in fried or sugary foods, or heavy drinking.

I am reminded of a middle-aged man who consumed half a dozen cans of diet soda a day, hardly exercised save for some periodic rock climbing, and snacked on junk food while at work. He told me one day that the results of some test, from his physical, impressed his doctor. I don't recall if it was the cholesterol test or high blood pressure test, or some other diagnostic test. But I quote this man as stating, "My doctor told me that whatever I'm doing, to keep on doing it!"

What this means is keep on filling his body with soda, artificial sweeteners and junk from vending machines. So maybe his test results came out normal. But how long before things start plummeting downhill for this man? The human body can take only so much abuse before it retaliates.

One thing I believe people need to grasp is the concept that illness and disease can take many years to manifest in the form of symptoms. Research indicates that heart disease begins during our teenage years and progresses from there. It may take 30, 40 or even 50 years before symptoms appear, prompting the patient to see a doctor. In the meantime, this patient's doctor has been proclaiming him or her "healthy" during routine visits *due to the absence of symptoms*.

But sooner or later it becomes "crisis management" time and the patient is told to start eating better, exercise more and is put on expensive and potentially dangerous statin drugs for the remainder of his or her life. The patient may also be sent for risky tests such as an angiogram and advised to undergo other cardiac procedures.

The case with former President Clinton is a perfect example. Routine physical exams with some of the nation's top doctors failed to show any danger of heart disease. When he finally began experiencing symptoms, doctors found that his arteries were 90 percent blocked and that he required emergency quadruple bypass surgery in order to save his life! Again, the absence of disease or pain should not be used as an indicator of an individual's true health status.

Every emotion we feel and every thought we have is a physical event. Although negative thoughts and emotions alone may not cause illness, they do affect us physically by triggering responses in the body that lead to chemical, hormonal, neurologic and molecular changes, which in turn allow sickness to flourish.

For example, when we are under stress, our body releases the stress hormone cortisol. High levels of cortisol can also raise heart rate and increase blood pressure and cholesterol levels. Cortisol also appears to play a role in the accumulation of abdominal fat and can lead to over-weight and obesity. Stress can also worsen many skin conditions—such as psoriasis, eczema, hives and acne. All of these setbacks may lead to depression, low self-esteem and social isolation, all of which may adversely affect the course of the conditions.

A Positive Outlook on Heart Disease

A growing body of research identifies a link between optimism and physical health. According to a study published in the *Journal of Psychosomatic Medicine*, optimism appears to reduce the risk of coronary heart disease in men. Having a positive outlook on life is the first step in reducing your risk of developing this deadly killer.

If your mind is consumed by unpleasant thoughts and feelings on a daily basis, you must make a conscious effort to rid yourself of these destructive forces. If left unchallenged, these negative thoughts will, without a doubt, increase your risk for depression and other physical ailments; and may reduce your life expectancy by as much as eight years. This is regardless of how many vitamins you take, how nutritiously you eat or how much you hit the gym.

Become an Optimist

Because of the clear benefits of adapting and maintaining a positive mental attitude, the first step in my longevity plan involves improving the health of your mind by becoming an optimist. Learning to become an optimist requires that you get into the habit of thinking positively, no matter how bad the situation may seem.

Generally speaking, optimists tend to:

- Be very specific in their descriptions, while pessimists tend to generalize. For example, a pessimist might use the expression, "Doctors are inconsiderate," while an optimist might say, "My doctor is inconsiderate."

- Have hope, while pessimists feel hopeless. Pessimists believe they are helpless in situations; doomed if they try; are more likely to suffer from stress, anxiety and depression; and are more likely to collapse under pressure.

- Blame factors beyond their control as the cause of their misfortune or failure, while pessimists blame themselves for their failures. This causes pessimists to have low self-esteem.

- View unpleasant events or challenges as temporary, while pessimists tend to believe negative situations will last a long time. A pessimist may give up, while an optimist will try hard to change the situation.

Next time you're about to face a tough task, don't think, "This is going to be difficult." Instead, think, "This is going to be challenging." Science has proven that we can consciously alter our brain responses and condition ourselves to think more positively. Thus, even if you tend to be the type of person who sees the bleakness in everything, you can break the habit with a little practice and learn to be an affirmative and optimistic thinker, all the time.

Each day when we awaken, we can choose to be either the masters or victims of our attitude. The person we are today is a result of the choices we've made yesterday. The person we are tomorrow will be a result of our outlook today.

I have encountered many people in my practice who have convinced themselves that they will never be healthy. They go to bed at night anticipating how worthless tomorrow will be. Not surprisingly, next morning they usually feel down and out, if not worse, than they did the previous day. Unhelpful thoughts weaken their immune systems and allow illness to breed within their bodies.

The first step in my plan lays the foundation for the other phases by helping change your thoughts and feelings and maintaining a positive mental attitude. As you work on this first phase, monitor your thoughts for old habits. Awareness of current patterns and behaviors will help you make permanent change to your mental attitude. When a habitual negative response starts to kick in, recall the way optimists tend to respond to such situations, and consciously redirect your mental processes toward uplifting responses.

Improve Your Attitude and Emotional Well-Being

The following techniques will help improve the health of your mind, and in turn, your body. In order to be effective, they must be practiced on a daily basis. Changing habitual behaviors does not happen overnight. It takes three weeks to start changing an old habit. You may wish to work on one technique per day, phasing in a new one as you progress. This will allow you to implement and monitor one change while maintaining any previous changes.

1. **Remove yourself from negativity.** You must extract yourself from down-and-out people and/or situations to develop and maintain a positive train of thought. Like that old saying goes: *You are whom you associate with.* If you hang out with downbeat people, their negative energy will rub off onto you. If you are healthy and surround yourself with people who always gripe about their illnesses, you are more likely to develop a discouraging view towards your own health and, subsequently, become sick. You may need to make some choices about your friends, colleagues and spouse if they are sources for negativity. A job change, transfer, separation or distance will help you avoid negativity from these people.

2. **Surround yourself with positivism.** As the saying goes, "Birds of a feather flock together." Individuals who are successful tend to surround themselves with others who are successful. There's an adage: *If*

you want to learn how to become rich, then hang out with rich folks. The same goes for being physically fit. Hang out with those who are full of energy and rarely suffer aches and pains. Surrounding yourself with positivism will help cleanse you of unfavorable thoughts and emotions and immediately give you a healthier outlook.

3. Control subconscious thoughts. We all tend to engage in "self-talk." When waiting to see the dentist, for instance, most of us probably think to ourselves, "I know this is going to be a painful experience," or when taking an exam we may reflect, "This is going to be hard. There's no way I'm ever going to pass." Self-deprecating thoughts typically develop into negative actions. Concentrate your energy on controlling negative self-talk and replace it with positive statements. People who think positively make an active attempt to block out these undesirable thoughts and consciously make an effort to imprint upbeat feelings in their subconscious mind. You can do it, too.

4. Believe in what you do. In order to be healthy you must truly believe that everything you do is a contributing factor to your health. To truly benefit from a positive attitude and outlook, you must sub-consciously believe that it will have a significant impact on the overall function of your immune system. The best example of this is the placebo effect described earlier. Each of us, whether sick or healthy, has the ability to tap into this power and improve our health dramatically. Even if you don't see results quickly, or continue to feel sick or unhealthy, believe that the positive changes you are implementing are working to make you better.

5. Practice positive affirmations and visualizations. An affirmation is a statement backed by emotional intensity. Positive affirmations help create a positive self-image. Examples of positive affirmations might include statements such as, "I am a healthy and energetic individual," or, "My body is a self-healing entity that has the power to overcome all illness and disease." Affirmations should always be positive and reflect the present tense. For a positive assertion to be effective, you must actually believe it to be true. Write several assertions for yourself and repeat them often throughout the day. The more often you repeat your positive declarations, the easier it will be to convince your mind they are reality. If you are ill and wish to become healthy, you must visualize yourself in a healthy state. Practicing positive visualizations can have a profound effect on our health. Set aside a specific time each day to review your positive visualizations. Close your eyes and see yourself sprinting along a beach or hoisting heavy garbage bags with ease. See yourself glowing with good health and happiness, doing all the things you enjoy.

6. Ask the right questions. Author and motivational speaker Tony Robbins believes that the quality of your life is equal to the quality of questions you ask yourself. According to Robbins, our brains will answer any questions asked of them. So a person who is suffering from a chronic illness or debilitating disease might continually ask herself, "Why do I always feel so bad," or, "Why can't I ever have a good day?" These types of questions destroy one's self-esteem and lead to feelings of helplessness, hopelessness and worthlessness. Asking yourself a higher quality question such as, "What can I do to improve the way I feel?" helps build
self-confidence and gives you a sense of control over the situation. By forcing your mind to answer questions that build self-might, you are inadvertently reprogramming your brain to think positively. The same can also be said of our attitudes toward aging. Many of us have the attitude that aging predisposes us to illness and disability. The older we get, the more negative our thoughts and emotions become. This, in turn, weakens our immune systems and ultimately creates an ideal environment for illness to fester. Listen to the questions you are asking and reframe them so that your mental attitude's default resets to "positive."

7. Set positive and realistic goals. Setting both short-and long-term positive goals helps build strong self-esteem and sense of worth. Achieving your short-term goals can help improve the way you feel about yourself on a daily, weekly or monthly basis. Short-term goals should be easily attainable and help you work towards achieving long-term goals. For example, if your long-term goal is to lose 100 pounds, your short-term goals might be to lose 5 pounds per month for the next 12 months. Each month when you reach or exceed your goal of 5 pounds you feel a lofty sense of accomplishment and self-esteem. Whatever your goals are, it's important they be within reach. Setting unrealistic goals will only lead to failure.

8. View problems as challenges and opportunities. Problems are a part of life, and you never know when they will appear. People who believe that troubles are ruining their lives are really ruining their health. Instead, as you work on this technique, try viewing a problem as an opportunity, and that will help build your self-assuredness and improve overall health. Approach the next setback or challenge in a different, non-habitual manner. Instead of labeling it as a setback, stop to evaluate the situation and find the opportunity hidden in the circumstance. If your computer "freezes up," don't see the incident as an obstacle; see it as a chance to learn something about the computer by trying to fix it yourself.

9. Laugh and have fun. A good sense of humor enables you to see the funny side of things, making a bad situation tolerable and painless. Laughter has been shown to increase and improve the immune system. Read the comics, watch classic comedy shows, bookmark funny websites, listen to comedy routines on CD, read humorous books, talk to young children whose fresh perspectives on life are often quite amusing, and play in the snow, climb a tree, romp in a pile of leaves, splash in the water or fly a kite. If it's been awhile since you engaged in a favorite activity, head to your workshop, garage, gym, sewing machine or hobby room, and dive in again. Schedule time for fun, just as you schedule regular appointments with the doctor.

10. Learn to be a giver. People who are generous to others tend to be healthier and have a more optimistic outlook on life. When you put others before yourself, you forget about your own problems and focus on how you can offer solutions to others. Find ways to give on a regular basis. You can give time by volunteering in many ways. Your community newspaper probably lists many places to volunteer. Help at your child's school, record books for the blind or start your own giving campaign for your favorite organization or cause. Take the focus off yourself, and your mental attitude will begin to soar. For individuals suffering from severe depression, grief, hopelessness or anxiety, I recommend seeking the help of a professional or joining a group support program. Keep in mind however, that none of these techniques will provide much benefit without first having a positive outlook towards your health.

Additional Tips to Improve the Health of Your Mind

1. **Exercise:** Aerobic exercise is an effective treatment for depression. It works, in part, by stimulating the release of endorphins that can improve mood. Walk, jog, skate or bike-ride for a pick-me-up.

2. **Breathing exercises:** Practicing the deep breathing exercises described in Chapter 3 can help release foul thoughts and emotions from the body and enhance your mood.

3. **Omega-3 fatty acids:** DHA, one of the omega-3s, is the main constituent of cell membranes in the brain. Dietary deficiencies of DHA have been implicated in bipolar disorder and depression. People with higher levels of omega-3 fatty acids in their blood were less likely to report mild-to-moderate depression, according to a recent study presented at the annual meeting of the American Psychosomatic Society. See the supplement chapter for proper dosing.

4   **St. John's wort for mild-to-moderate depression:** To help boost your mood, take 900 mg per day, divided into three doses. Results may take up to six weeks.

5. **5-HTP for mild-to-moderate depression:** 5-HTP (L-5-hydroxy-tryptophan) is derived from griffonia (griffonia simplicifolia) seeds, and is the immediate precursor to serotonin, the brain nutrient for relaxation. Numerous clinical trials have studied the efficacy of 5-HTP for treating depression. One compared 5-HTP to the antidepressant drug fluvoxamine and found 5-HTP to be equally effective. The effective dose of 5-HTP appears to be between 50 and 500 mg daily. Used in combination with other antidepressant substances, however, the effective dose may be even lower. Research shows that some people respond better to lower doses, so I recommend beginning at the low end of the dose range and increasing as necessary. 5-HTP may not be appropriate for all types of depression and may not be compatible with all types of medication. Consultation with a health care practitioner is strongly advised.

6.   **Ginkgo biloba:** Conditions such as depression, anxiety and age-related dementia have all been linked to reduced blood flow to the brain. By improving blood circulation, ginkgo may be useful for treating these disorders, especially in older people. For depression, the recommended dose is 240 mg of ginkgo biloba extract (GBE) per day. GBE supplements should contain at least 24 percent flavone glycosides (to maximize the herb's antioxidant and anti-clotting potential), and 6 percent terpene lactones (for improved blood flow and nerve protection).

Senior Wasteland

I was once in a major chain home improvement store, and as I walked through the door, saw an elderly man smiling and waving at everyone entering. He was employed as a greeter and was very frail-looking with a slumped posture. Most people would think it was "cute," even admirable, that he was working such a job, "keeping active." Regardless of whether or not they are doing it for financial reasons, I always wonder, "What type of lifestyle did this person lead during their early years and even at their current age?"

If a person spends 40 hours a week as a greeter (or some other similar job) in the name of "doing something," this will interfere with opportunities to provide ample stimulation to the brain cells. You cannot sprout new neural connections by waving your hand like a robot and sounding like a broken record, "Hi, how are you? Hi, how are you?"

The retired person will get more brain cell and physical stimulation if he or she does NOT take a job such as school bus driver, custodian, grocery sacker, and the proverbial department store greeter, and instead keeps busy with a variety of activities (analogous to eating a variety of fruits and vegetables rather than just the same food all the time); activities that force the brain cells into action, and the cardiorespiratory and musculoskeletal systems into action.

That 40-hours-a-week, spent adhering to the boss's schedule, can instead be used up with the following activities (assuming the person is financially comfortable, and many senior greeters or checkout clerks actually are quite financially comfortable with their previous job's pension):

- Lessons in oil or water color painting, pottery, drawing, print-making, sculpture
- Lessons with a musical instrument
- Lessons in yoga, tai chi, martial arts (yes, seniors can benefit tremendously from this art form; instruction is based on individual ability), weight training
- Attending aerobics, dance or swimming classes
- Joining a group for walkers, hikers, cyclists
- Joining a bowling league
- Learning a second language, reading classic literature, attending symphonies, taking computer, astronomy or philosophy classes at the local college, cultivating a garden
- Volunteering for environmental causes, animal causes, children's causes, political causes

Gee, this barely leaves a little time to visit the grandkids! But of course, that should never be neglected. When a person fills his or her life with an abundance of intellectually, creatively and physically stimulating pursuits, this will more profoundly give rise to a stronger, fitter body and longer life span, than standing in virtually one spot for hours on end, greeting customers, or tapping endlessly on a cash register, or hunched over the steering wheel of a bus.

This brings to mind the very old-looking man who spent hours in a shed-like structure, in the parking lot of a major auto dealership. His job was to hand the keys back to customers who had their cars serviced; the customer would give him paperwork, and he'd fetch the corresponding keys. And that was it.

Now, maybe he desperately needed the money. But there's a good chance that he was working to "get out of the house," or to "keep active." Unfortunately, the activity was sitting on a stool all day, and not a whole lot of brain cells were needed to conduct this job. The man looked decrepit, with arthritic, gnarled hands, and loads of deep crevices in his face.

Obviously, he was no candidate for the local senior basketball league, but it's not difficult to imagine the serious upgrades in his physical and mental state that would have resulted had he never gotten that job, and instead, filled his days with some of the activities named above.

I went there for an oil change one day and noticed the shed was gone, and so was the man. I wonder if he died. But I needn't wonder how much better his health would have been, had he spent his time involved with more challenging tasks.

A common argument is, "Hey, if he likes what he does, why criticize it? Maybe he enjoys it!" This man never cracked the slightest smile. But don't let that fool you. It's very possible that he wanted this job, in the name of either getting out of the house, getting away from his wife, or having "something to do," even though it wasn't enough to produce any smiles. How sad that this man represents many older people who don't realize what kind of options exist for charging up their mind and body.

The argument of, "If that's what he wants to do, then what's wrong with it?" can also be applied to a two-pack-a-day smoker who lives on fast-food. If that's what makes him happy, why fault it? If your daughter were a heavy smoker and ate nothing but junk food, and she told you, "But it makes me happy!" would this be of any consolation to you?

Bottom line: Our brains and bodies should be richly stimulated right to our graves.

In a Nutshell

One of the most compelling and intriguing examples of the power of the mind to heal is the placebo effect. Think about it…you are told by your doctor that you have an untreatable form of cancer. Your doctor then informs you that you have the option of trying an experimental drug designed to treat your specific cancer. You agree and begin taking the "drug." Amazingly, you begin to feel better and your condition improves. You improve to the point that there is no longer evidence of cancer in your body. You are then told that you were merely given a sugar pill and not the cancer drug that the others in the study were given.

This phenomenon occurs commonly in many drug trials—where both groups of subjects (those given the actual medication and those given the sugar pills) actually improve equally. So what is the explanation for this? We all know that a sugar pill is not capable of healing an individual from a specific illness or disease. What actually improved or healed the individual's illness was the faith they had in the pill (sugar) they were given. In other words, the individual truly believed in their mind that the pill they were taking could improve or cure their body. This is the healing power of the mind at work. The mind-body connection to health has been well-documented in the scientific literature.

Negative or self-deprecating thoughts, emotions and attitudes wreak havoc on the body. The result? Signals are sent from our brain that depress the immune system and increase your vulnerability to crippling illness and disease.

On the other hand, many good-natured, cheerful thoughts, positive emotions and an upbeat attitude actually strengthen the activity of the immune system and will help your body remain healthy, and/or assist in healing from injury and recovering from illness.

Research indicates that optimists live an average of 10 years longer than pessimists. Yes, that's right. Change your attitude and you will add an additional 10 years to your life! Wake up each day and tell yourself that it's going to be a good day (or a better day than yesterday), and with time, your body will begin to reward you with better health.

Chapter 2 Goals:

- ✓ Change negative thoughts, emotions and attitudes to hopeful and optimistic ones.
- ✓ Truly believe that your body is a self-healing mechanism and that every positive lifestyle change you make (healthy diet, exercise, supplementation, rest, etc.) is positively influencing your health and your body's ability to fend off illness and disease.
- ✓ Associate with cheerful, upbeat people. Avoid negative, critical people as much as possible.

Chapter 3

Is Stress Killing You?

Life Extension Value: 17 years

Top Ten Stressors

1. Death of spouse
2. Divorce
3. Marital separation
4. Jail term
5. Death of close family member
6. Personal injury or illness
7. Marriage
8. Fired at work
9. Marital reconciliation
10. Retirement

Stress and Your Life

Some days you probably think that your anxiety is engulfing you—and you are right. Stress is a serious health problem, and according to medical researchers, 75-90 percent of all visits to primary care physicians are for complaints and conditions that are, in some way, stress-related. Every week, over 115 million people take some form of medication for stress-related symptoms.

The workplace is a major source of stress. You have to wonder if a person really means it when he or she says, "I love my job!" Maybe people make this proclamation rather than admit that, deep down, they really hate their job. More heart attacks occur on Mondays than any other day of the week. Coincidence? For many people, their job is synonymous with sheer anxiety. That means that the body is subjected for 40 hours or more per week to factors that can alter the human machine's ability to properly function.

On the other hand, people staying at home most of the time may also face incredible stress. For a mother who lacks nurturing and organizational skills, it may be nerve-wrenching when everyone (including her husband) is crying for attention at the same time. For the perfectionist, a few crumbs on the cocktail table can send him or her into a frenzy. For a commuter who is already late for work, it might be simply catching another red light. Or for someone who has to work late at the office, it may mean having to miss a child's birthday party. The common thread: all of these situations are stressful.

Neurotics Don't Live Long

While genetics and lifestyle clearly play a major role in longevity, new research suggests that those who live to be 100 are less likely to dwell on problems, and have developed better coping mechanisms to deal with stress than those who die younger.

In a small study of women centenarians, researchers at Boston Medical Center in New England found low levels of neuroticism among the oldest people in the group. Neuroticism commonly includes symptoms of anxiety, obsessions and phobias. Additional studies involving centenarians around the world suggest that they have higher morale than other seniors, and that psychological health is more important than physical health in maintaining well-being late in life. According to Margery Silver, associate director of the New England study, "Centenarians are temperamentally natural stress managers, but the rest of us can learn ways to manage our stress." Centenarians in the study also tended to be funny and gregarious, and "able to build the kind of social networks that are important to cognitive vitality."

If you want to improve your health and increase your chances of a long and healthy life, you must develop effective coping mechanisms to deal with stress.

The Stress Response

Commonly called the "fight-or-flight" reaction, the stress response prepares the body to function at a higher level, thus increasing the chance for survival in a threatening situation. Imagine walking along a quiet street when suddenly, out of nowhere, a barking dog the size of a cheetah charges at you. You instantly feel a surge of adrenaline course through your body. Your heart and breathing rate increase rapidly, your muscles tense, blood sugar levels go up for energy, and blood is diverted to the extremities in an attempt to prepare the body for fight or flight.

It's estimated that the average person experiences nearly 50 stressors per day. Although these events aren't life-or-death situations, your body still responds to them with a "fight-or-flight" reaction. What happened to your body last time your boss at work said to you, "I need to see you in my office"?

Each time we encounter a stressor, the pituitary gland in the brain releases stress hormones, including **cortisol**, which is released in an attempt to reduce inflammation at the site of any potential wounds. The pituitary gland doesn't know that being called into your boss's office won't result in any physical wounds. The hormone gets pumped out anyways.

In excessive amounts, it can actually weaken the immune system and increase your susceptibility to disease. High levels of cortisol have also been linked to weight gain, digestive disorders, sleep disturbances and loss of sex drive. Other stress hormones trigger the release of fats into the bloodstream that increase cholesterol levels and may accelerate the buildup of fatty plaques within the arteries.

Researchers have found that individuals who have experienced several stressful events within a year have a much higher probability of developing a serious illness than non-stressed individuals. Once stress hormones are released into the bloodstream, they can remain active for a long time, causing considerable damage to the body.

Stress and Adrenal "Burnout"

The adrenal glands can also be damaged from chronic exposure to stress. Under stressful conditions, the adrenals are forced to work harder and eventually may "burn out." Symptoms of adrenal "burnout" include fatigue, nervousness and irritability, depression, muscle weakness, brittle nails, headaches, salt cravings, allergies, sparse body hair, poor memory and concentration skills, and frequent confusion.

Some ailments and illnesses linked to prolonged stress exposure

- Angina
- Asthma
- Autoimmune diseases
- Cancer
- Cardiovascular disease
- Chronic fatigue syndrome
- Common cold
- Depression
- Diabetes (Type II)
- Gastrointestinal disturbances
- Headaches
- High blood pressure
- Immune system compromise
- Insomnia
- Irritable bowel syndrome
- Menstrual irregularities
- Rheumatoid arthritis
- Stroke
- Ulcerative colitis
- Ulcers

Stress and Your Heart

In a major study appearing in the journal *Lancet*, researchers surveyed more than 11,000 heart-attack victims and found that in the year prior to their attacks, they had been under significantly more stress than a control group of 13,000 healthy individuals. Stress was determined to be comparable to risk factors such as high blood pressure and abdominal obesity, even though variables such as diet and exercise were considered.

Stress management is essential in the prevention of heart disease. In fact, it's just as important as other factors such as a healthy diet and regular exercise. "Diet and exercise alone are like a two-legged stool," says Dr. Redford Williams, director of the Behavior Medicine Research Center at Duke University. "It's more stable with the third leg: stress management."

Stress and Diabetes

Stress hormones lead to an increase in the amount of glucose (sugar) in the blood. Because diabetics are unable to produce enough insulin to metabolize the increased sugar in the blood, it remains high long after the stress has ended. Over time, chronically high or heavily fluctuating blood sugar levels can inflict enormous hidden damage to the body.

Stress and Digestive Disorders

You have just closed your car door and realize that your keys are inside. Your gut clenches and you immediately begin to feel frazzled and queasy. One in four people today seek treatment for a gastrointestinal problem such as heartburn or irritable bowel syndrome (IBS). Upon examination, most of these people have normal blood tests and abdominal X-rays. **But the absence of positive diagnostic findings does not mean that nothing is wrong.**

The brain and digestive system communicate through a common network that emotional unrest can disrupt. Stress-related digestive problems commonly defy conventional treatments. If the stress is not managed, the disorders will typically become progressively worse or not improve.

Evaluating Stress

It would be nice if you could go to your doctor to get a specific test to detect your current level of stress, and use the test results to help determine your risk for developing a particular disease. Unfortunately, at this time, there is no such exam.

However, several self-assessment tests are available to help you evaluate the amount of stress, hidden stress and potential pressures in your life. Two of these tests are included in Appendix A of this publication.

Symptoms of Stress Overload

Symptoms of stress overload can vary among individuals. In some people, stress may lead to headaches, sleep disturbances or concentration problems, while in others it can result in depression, bigger appetite, irregular heartbeat, chest pains, gastrointestinal problems and/or muscle tension and aches.

Because stress can compromise resistance to illness, individuals under chronic angst may also experience frequent colds and infections. Over time, stress overload can increase an individual's risk for serious sickness and/or disease, including cardiovascular disorders and cancer. Research has shown that individuals suffering from serious illness have a better chance at recovery when they implement a successful stress management plan.

The Relaxation Response

The mirror image of the "stress" response is the "relaxation response," identified by Dr. Herbert Benson in 1974. While studying a group of people practicing transcendental meditation, he observed specific physiological changes opposite those seen during the stress response.

The relaxation response appears to be an antidote to the effects of the stress reaction. The key to activating this response lies in the stimulation of the parasympathetic nervous system. When this system is stimulated through a rhythmical activity such as deep breathing patterns, meditation or the repetition of prayer, the individual will begin to experience a sense of calm and relaxation—leading to a reduction in blood pressure, perspiration, muscle tension and breathing rate, plus increased relaxation.

Practicing techniques that elicit the relaxation response has been found to enhance the effectiveness of the body's natural defenses and self-repair mechanisms. Other positive changes associated with the relaxation response include improved emotional well-being and better coping of nerve-jarring situations.

A variety of techniques can be used to elicit the relaxation response, most of which are the basis of mind/body medicine. Some of the more common techniques used to elicit this response include meditation, deep breathing exercises, progressive relaxation techniques, yoga and so on. Several of these methods are discussed in detail at the end of this section. Many can be practiced in the comfort of your home or office in only a few minutes.

Effective Stress Management

To successfully combat the effects of stress, you must first identify its primary sources. Truly make an attempt to eliminate or reduce your exposure to stressors. Negative coping patterns such as smoking, drinking and overeating must also be replaced with more constructive measures such as relaxation techniques (meditation and deep breathing), vigorous exercise, stretching exercises, listening to soothing music and holistic supplementation.

The recommendations and techniques described in the remainder of this chapter will help you to cope with stress and in turn, improve your overall health. Keep in mind that to be effective, they must be practiced consistently.

The Medical Alternative

Medical management of stress typically entails the use of pharmaceutical agents designed to relieve anxiety and tension. But these drugs have a host of undesirable, and sometimes deadly, side effects. At best, these drugs only mask the symptoms of stress rather than bolstering your body's ability to cope with it. If your doctor is unwilling to discuss natural alternatives, find one who is.

The Natural Alternative

Implementing the following changes into your life will help your body deal with the "fight or flight" response and will reduce the likelihood of stress-induced illness.

1. Dietary changes
2. Exercise
3. Nutritional support
4. Relaxation techniques
5. Time management skills

Dietary Changes

Dietary recommendations for stress management are simple. Increase your intake of whole, fresh fruits and vegetables, and healthy oils, while reducing consumption of fried and processed foods, refined carbohydrates, caffeine and alcohol. These recommendations are also the cornerstone of our life extension diet detailed in Chapter 3.

Regular Exercise

Routine exercise is an essential component of any stress management program. People who exercise on a consistent basis are much less likely to suffer from fatigue, anxiety and depression, and are better able to handle stressful situations than are sedentary individuals. People who work out are also much happier and less prone to suicide than their more inactive counterparts.

Ever notice on TV talk shows, whenever the guests are people who've struggled with all sorts of problems in life, from abusive relationships to having out-of-control teenagers, their bodies more often than not look as though they've never exercised a day in their life? Their posture is poor, they're frequently obese, or they are underweight with sunken chests and toothpick arms. They just don't look the least bit healthy. So which came first? The bad health, which then led to infidelity or troubles with their kids? Or did the bad circumstances hit first, then causing a decline in fitness?

Structured exercise trains the body to deal better with physical stress. This then carries over to being better equipped to face emotional stress—such as raising kids or holding down a job. You will rarely see people with the body of a marble statue sitting on a talk show crying about how their spouse batters them, how their 10-year-old hits them and behaves like a savage at school, or that their 13-year-old is sexually active. Coincidence? Or can exercise actually train the mind to be more disciplined? And that increased self-discipline would certainly carry over to all facets of life.

Habitually engaging in exercise causes an array of chemical changes in the brain, including those involved in mood enhancement. Exercise can stimulate production of **endorphins**. Endorphins are considered to be the body's natural painkillers and mood boosters, and are responsible for the "high" that many runners experience during a workout. Endorphins are similar in chemical structure to morphine. They naturally relieve pain and promote feelings of well-being and relaxation. Just 10 minutes of vigorous exercise can elevate endorphin levels for an hour after the activity has ended.

Exercise provides a feeling of self-worth and accomplishment. When a person feels this way, he or she is less likely to stay in an abusive relationship, and less likely to supply an environment to their kids that will give rise to rebellious behavior.

The best form of exercise for stress reduction involves activities that result in rhythmic physical exertion, such as swimming laps, brisk walking, jogging, bicycling and aerobics classes. These create a training effect. This training effect strengthens the heart and improves lung capacity. Additionally, the hormonal system and metabolic reactions are also strengthened in their ability to cope with stressors. In Chapter 5, I will help you design an effective exercise program that will reduce stress and improve your chances for optimal wellness.

Nutritional Support

Nutritional support for stress management typically involves supporting the adrenal glands. The nutrients important for this function are:

- Vitamin C
- B-complex
- Zinc
- Magnesium

Studies have shown the concentration of these nutrients to be less than optimal in individuals repeatedly exposed to high levels of stress. A vitamin C deficiency can weaken the immune system. Increased consumption of food rich in vitamin C and/or supplementation may be necessary to normalize blood levels during times of stress. *Dose: 60 mg per day, with optimal intake ranging from 500 to 1,000 mg daily.*

Under stress, the body's demand for B vitamins is also increased, especially vitamin B-5 (pantothenic acid) and B-6 (pyroxidine). B vitamins are essential for maintenance of nerve and brain cells. A vitamin B deficiency can result in adrenal shrinkage, and can lead to symptoms of fatigue, headache, insomnia, nausea and abdominal distress.

Herbal support for stress management typically includes kava and ginseng. Kava has been found to possess anti-anxiety properties similar to that of oxazepam (a drug similar to Valium) without the undesirable side effects. *Dose: 45-70 milligrams of kavalactones three times daily, or 135-210 mg of kavalactones as a single dose one hour before bedtime.* Kava should never be taken with anti-anxiety drugs like Prozac or alcohol, as the substances may multiply each other's effect.

Ginseng has been found to improve an individual's ability to cope with both physical and mental anguish. Ginseng works by delaying the onset and reducing the severity of the "fight or flight" response. Clinical studies have shown ginseng to be equally as effective as Valium in reducing the feeling of anxiety, without the side effects. *Dose: 1-2 grams of crude ginseng root three times daily, or 100 mg one to three times daily of standardized extract containing 5 percent ginsenosides.* The Chinese (Panax) variety of ginseng is generally regarded as the most potent.

Relaxation Therapies

The primary goal of relaxation therapies is to allow the individual to achieve a sense of relaxation by tapping the inner power of the mind and body. Many of these therapies focus on the repetition of a specific sound, word or prayer, which in turn, induces relaxation and mops up stress. When practiced regularly, relaxation therapies can help enhance immune function and improve the body's ability to combat stress and recover from illness.

While you're in a state of relaxation, brain waves slow, respiration decreases, and the utilization of oxygen by the body is reduced by 20 percent. Heart rate and blood pressure also decrease. Relaxation therapies have been used successfully to treat a variety of medical ills.

Some popular forms of relaxation therapy: meditation, yoga, t'ai chi, deep breathing, progressive muscle relaxation, guided imagery, biofeedback and humor. These therapies can be used alone or in conjunction with medication and/or surgery. To be effective, relaxation techniques must be practiced on a regular basis.

Rather than go into detail about each of these techniques, I have chosen to focus on meditation, deep breathing exercises and humor therapy. These highly effective techniques are simple to learn, can be performed almost anywhere and require no special training or equipment.

Meditation

Meditation can be broadly defined as any activity that keeps the attention pleasantly anchored in the present moment. There are four elements common to most forms of meditation: a quiet and peaceful environment; a comfortable body posture; something to focus on like an object, a word or breathing; and a passive, receptive attitude. Meditation typically requires 10-30 minutes, and is most effective when practiced daily.

Regular practice of meditation can help reduce blood pressure, heart rate, respiration, anxiety and pain levels. An 18-year study published in the *American Journal of Cardiology* (2005) claims that practicing meditation can extend people's life span and reduce risk of dying from cardiovascular disease or cancer. Researchers found that those who practiced meditation had a 23 percent reduction in overall death rate, a 30 percent reduction in cardiovascular disease death rate, and a 49 percent reduction in cancer death rate, when compared to those not practicing meditation.

Below is a simple technique that can be used to meditate, and thus elicit the relaxation response. The two basic components necessary to achieve this response is a mantra, a single word or syllable that is repeated over and over in a rhythmic, chant-like manner (silently or aloud), and the disregard of other thoughts that come to mind during the mantra.

1. Find a quiet, comfortable place to sit or lie and close your eyes.
2. Relax all your muscles.
3. Breathing through your nose, repeat silently or aloud a mantra every time you exhale.

4. When disruptive thoughts enter your mind, let them go and return to your mantra. The more you practice, the longer you'll stay focused.
5. Continue for 10-20 minutes.
6. Attempt to meditate once in the morning and again later in the day.

Deep Breathing

Under stressful situations, our breathing patterns become more rapid and shallow, heart rate increases and the muscles in the body become tense. When most adults breathe, they tend to fill only their upper chest with air, a sign of shallow breathing. Chest breathing is similar to the type of breathing induced during the "fight or flight" stress response.

Over time, the body can create the edgy feelings associated with that response. Deep breathing slows heart rate, dilates blood vessels and relaxes muscles. It is also thought to improve symptoms of depression, as it has a relaxing effect on the mind. Taking fuller breaths also provides the body with a greater supply of energy, which can be used to fuel the body's self-repair mechanisms.

The deep breathing exercise listed below can help improve your breathing and provide you with wonderful benefits. This technique involves the use of the diaphragm to breathe, which alters a person's physiology by activating the relaxation center in the brain.

1. Sit or lie comfortably in a quiet place.
2. With your feet slightly apart, place one hand on your abdomen near your navel, and the other hand on your chest.
3. Inhale through your nose and exhale through your mouth, concentrating on your breathing pattern.
4. Inhale while slowly counting to 4. As you exhale, slightly extend your abdomen, causing it to rise about one inch. You should initially feel your abdomen rise, then your chest as it fills with air.
5. As you breathe in, imagine warm or cool air flowing in and going to all parts of your body.
6. Pause for one second, then exhale slowly to a count of 4. You should notice your abdomen moving inward as you exhale.

7. As you exhale, imagine all the tension and stress leaving your body.
8. Continue this process for about 10-15 minutes.
9. Resume normal breathing if you feel faint or lightheaded.

Humor Therapy

Studies conducted at Loma Linda University School of Medicine in California have found that laughter stimulates the immune system. Students who watched comedy videos had significant increases in T cells and natural killer cells, both of which fight off diseases. They also had lower levels of cortisol in their blood.

In a second study involving 240 heart attack victims, researchers at the Oakhurst Health Research Institute found that those who spent 30 minutes a day watching comedy videos were less likely to suffer a second heart attack.

Ways to incorporate humor therapy into your life:

■ Watch comedy shows, films and videos regularly.
■ Read a funny book or story daily.
■ Spend time with friends or family members who make you laugh.
■ Put yourself in the company of children, who almost always evoke laughter.

Reduce Stress with Improved Time Management Skills

Poor time management is one of the biggest stressors we face. Like that old saying goes: Lost time is never found. The constant feeling of never having enough time to get things done can cause a lot of torment. Effective time management will help reduce this. Below are some time-managing tips.

1. **Set realistic goals and expectations—in both the workplace and personal relationships.** As our lives become busier, we have less and less time to devote to our own well-being. Establishing realistic expectations involves knowing your limits and feeling comfortable saying "no" to demands you cannot meet. Rather than always trying to "get the job done," priori-

tize your responsibilities. Handle your most important priorities first, leaving the busywork for later in the day.

2. **Stop procrastinating.** Putting things off only creates more work at a later time. Make a list of the day's tasks the night before, and tackle first the most important. The unimportant ones can wait. Also avoid putting off the unpleasant tasks, which tend to increase stress levels when we think of them.

3. **Give yourself adequate time when traveling.** Just the thought of being late can release stress hormones. Allow yourself additional time when traveling and accept the fact that traffic delays are part of your daily schedule. Make the most of traffic time by practicing relaxation techniques. Listening to soft music in your car can also calm the mind and body. Anger and frustration will not take you to your destination any sooner. They'll only increase stress levels and possibly make you crash your car into a light post...a sure way to shorten life span!

4. **Avoid being a perfectionist.** Spending countless hours on a specific project will only delay the completion of others, leading to an abundance of work later on. Try doing the best job possible in a reasonable amount of time, and then move on to the next task. If you have additional time, go back and polish up your work.

5. **Make time for yourself.** Break away from your busy schedule, even if for only a few minutes, to take a short walk, stretch your body, read a book or favorite magazine, listen to music, play a game, enjoy a cup of herbal tea or have a few laughs with a friend or loved-one.

6. **Accept circumstances you cannot change:** Many issues that cause distress are beyond our control, such as traffic jams and accidents, car problems and airline delays. Try to recognize and accept these situations, as they are a part of life for most of us.

Keep these tips in mind to help you adopt the "I can" frame of mind:

- Focus on the things you can change and accomplish.
- Stop worrying about things you cannot control.
- Start each day with a positive attitude.
- Find contentment in what you do.
- Find creative solutions to problems.
- Look for the positive, and not the negative, in other people.

Once you accept your stress for what it really is, you can take steps to control it.

> Stress has been linked to three of our nation's top killers: heart disease, stroke and cancer. Depression and anxiety, which afflict millions of Americans, can be caused or worsened by stress. It may also trigger flare-ups of asthma, rheumatoid arthritis and/or gastrointestinal disorders such as irritable bowel syndrome, colitis or peptic ulcers.

In a Nutshell

Studies have estimated that 75-90 percent of all visits to primary care physicians are for complaints and conditions that are, in some way, stress-related. Some conditions linked to stress include the common cold, high blood pressure, gastrointestinal disturbances, insomnia, cardiovascular disease and even cancer. Chronic exposure to stress can make us ill and lead to a premature death.

Although it's impossible to avoid stress altogether, it is possible to improve the way you cope or deal with stress. There are some people who become unhinged if their spouse leaves dirty socks on the floor of their magnificent home; and yet, there are other people who remain calm and collected through a hurricane that destroys their dream house. The second type of person will have far fewer stress toxins rampaging throughout his or her body, despite suffering the loss of their home; whereas, the first type of individual will experience greatly increased risk of disease, due to self-induced levels of stress disrupting his or her immune system.

Do you freak out if your child drops food on the floor? Or do you simply, and calmly, wipe it up—or better yet, casually instruct your child (if old enough), to help clean it up? It's not the stress that happens to you that counts; it's how you respond to it.

To successfully control stress, you must first identify its primary sources and make an attempt to eliminate or reduce your exposure to stressors. In situations where it's impossible to eliminate a cause of stress (traffic jams, loss of a job, death of a family member, etc.), one must develop effective methods for coping. Remember, stress itself is not harmful to the body. It's the way we react to it that matters most.

Negative coping patterns such as binging, drinking, smoking and overreacting must be replaced with more constructive measures such as relaxation techniques (deep breathing, progressive relaxation), lifestyle modification, exercise, proper diet, holistic supplementation—and even keeping a diary can soothe the harried soul. Doing so will help reduce the harmful effects of stress on the body and help improve health and well-being.

I offer several very simple yet effective methods for handling stress in this chapter. Best of all, these techniques take just a few minutes each day (10-15 min.) and will do wonders for your overall health. Make a commitment to spend a few minutes each day practicing one or more of these techniques, especially deep breathing exercises and meditation.

An 18-year study published in the *American Journal of Cardiology* (2005) found that practicing meditation can reduce your overall risk of death by 23 percent. If we assume the average life expectancy for humans is about 77 years, a 23% increase would amount to a difference of about 17 years. You decide if it's worth the 10-15 minutes a day.

Chapter 3 Goals

✓ Identify the primary sources of stress in your life.
✓ Make an attempt to reduce or eliminate exposure to common stressors.
✓ Replace negative coping patterns such as smoking, drinking and overeating with more constructive measures such as relaxation techniques, vigorous exercise, stretching exercises, and holistic supplementation.
✓ Practice the deep breathing exercises described in this chapter daily for a minimum of 10 minutes to help combat stress. Meditation is also an acceptable alternative, but can be more demanding in terms of time and focus.

Chapter 4

The Longevity Diet—12 Foods That Can Extend Your Life

Life Extension Value: 30 Years

"One should eat to live, not live to eat." Cicero

Our busy lives have led us to eating on the run, which ultimately leads to consumption of heavily processed fried and fast-foods, or sugary junk items. But even non-busy people will eat a junk-based diet; imagine how tempting this is when one spends hours every day watching TV, playing on the computer or talking on the phone. Boredom gives rise to eating for the wrong reasons.

We spend extra at the gas pump for high octane fuel, then head inside the shop to buy some "low octane" fuel to cram down our throats. Is there such a thing as a gas station that *doesn't* have some advertisement posted right above the gas pump—complete with huge photos—for some great bargain for a super-sized soda and a chili cheese dog or donuts? And let's face it: Those photos of the donuts are so vivid, your mouth waters just staring at them. The diet industry racks up a fortune every year from Americans on the weight-loss bandwagon. Yet 64 percent of U.S. adults remain either overweight or obese—the highest incidence on the planet.

What we should be eating has been rather hotly debated in the recent past. Current research in the field of nutritional science has taught us that a diet high in refined carbohydrates can trigger the early onset of Type 2 diabetes and fosters heart disease. The constant barrage of research telling us that something once believed healthy now causes cancer or some other serious disease further adds to the bewilderment.

> According to the US Surgeon General's Report on Nutrition and Health, 75 percent of cardiovascular disease, 60 percent of women's cancers, and 40 percent of men's cancers are related to nutrition and diet.

So who is right and what should we really be eating to optimize our health and increase our chances of longevity? Most people understand what they should *not* be eating (but many eat harmful foods anyways). If the poor choices are more or less obvious, what are the good choices when it comes to what you should feed your body?

If you're like most people, you're not interested in attending weekly meetings, counting calories, measuring portions, classifying foods into various groups and determining your blood or metabolic type when it comes to eating.

- Eating should be a pleasure, not a guilt-provoking drudgery that requires mathematical calculations.
- Think of food as sustenance, not as something to get all worked up about.
- Reflect upon how early mankind regarded food: as a fuel source to sustain an active body.

The ideal "diet" should be simple to understand and follow, and offer all the benefits of a healthful diet. My longevity plan is just that: a simple guide to eating well that will yield numerous long-term health benefits that those other plans just can't deliver. It harbors the synergistic effects of "superfoods" that have been proven to supercharge the body's defense system against an array of illnesses and diseases.

My longevity diet is not a "diet" per se, but a lifetime way of eating that promotes optimal health and longevity. It will give you the best possible shot at life extension and optimal health if followed religiously. My eating plan is based on the disease-preventative powers of the Mediterranean; characterized by foods rich in omega-3 fatty acids,

fresh fruits and vegetables, legumes, nuts, and whole grains, and copi-
ous amounts of olive oil.

There is an abundance of epidemiological evidence suggesting that
the Mediterranean diet can significantly reduce the risk for cardiovascular disease and cancer, and increase life span. My plan takes the traditional Mediterranean diet one step further and actually emphasizes
the intake of specific foods and drinks that have been proven to offer
the highest level of protection from our nation's deadliest killers.

This eating plan is based on the latest research including data from
the Harvard Nurses' Health Study, the Physicians' Health Study, and
the Health Professionals Follow-Up Study. The plan requires that you
understand your choices, and guides you toward making better
choices about what you eat and how you eat it.

Whom this eating plan is for:

- People wanting to maximize their life span and who plan on
  one day playing in the yard with their great-grandkids
- People who currently suffer from illness or disease and want to
  give their body the best chance at recovery and better health
- People who can't stick to a weight-loss diet
- People struggling with appetite control
- People who are utterly confused about what they should and
  should not eat
- People who lack energy

Benefits of the Longevity Diet:

- Significant protection against the onset of heart disease and
  stroke
- Significant protection against many types of cancer
- Protection against the onset of Type 2 diabetes
- Loss of excess body fat
- Improved gastrointestinal health
- Improved brain function
- Younger and healthier looking skin and hair
- Protection against premature aging

The Longevity Diet

The Longevity Diet requires little effort beyond willpower and some common sense when it comes to meal planning. I designed the plan for simplicity.

1. Increase intake of plant foods. Plant foods such as whole grains, fruits and vegetables, nuts and legumes, should compromise the majority of your daily food volume.
2. Reduce consumption of animal products. Restrict protein to certain types of fish, lean free-range meats and poultry, and eggs. Consume fatty fish, red meats and dairy products **only sparingly**.
3. Increase intake of dietary fiber.
4. Increase and balance ratio of healthy fats, especially omega-3s.
5. Restrict intake of sugar and refined carbohydrates.
6. Eat less, but more often.
7. Consume only clean water. Avoid unfiltered tap water.
8. Limit foods containing artificial additives, chemical dyes, preservatives and fake sweeteners. The closer to nature a food is, the better it is for you. The same holds true for beverages.

More Plant Foods

The low-carb diet revolution has convinced many people that carbs are bad and that a diet rich in red meat and fat provides the path to a fit and healthy body. Unfortunately, most people following these diets are not seeing the complete picture, and endanger their health in the process. Increasing your intake of protein and fat may yield the short-term benefit of temporary weight loss (most of which is water), but ultimately, will increase your risk for numerous diseases.

By omitting or restricting the intake of certain foods or food groups, namely complex carbohydrates, from your diet, deficiencies in key nutrients and antioxidants will develop over time. People who choose a low-carb diet eliminate nature's answer to great health: plant foods. Plant foods are low in calories, fat, and sodium and contain no cholesterol. They are also rich in vitamins and minerals, essential fatty acids, antioxidants and fiber. Additionally, plant foods contain thousands of different protective phytonutrients (*phyto* means plant) that help fend off disease.

The only protective nutrient that has been identified in animal products is omega-3 fatty acids. Animal products also contain high amounts of saturated fat and cholesterol. You can even see the harmful fat on the food itself: Check out any raw cut of steak. But have you ever seen gobs of sticky white fat on fruit, beans or greens? You may cut away the meat fat, but there's still plenty of it intertwined all throughout the cut, and your shearing knife will never get it all.

Many people falsely assume that a healthy diet requires daily meat consumption, the "meat and potatoes" mindset. Even one fast-food empire once ran a campaign for their burgers and fries, dubbing them, "America's meat and potatoes." (*Whole* potatoes are actually a healthy food, but not when they are fried and soaked in saturated fat oils.)

The truth is, our bodies are more than capable of remaining healthy on a plant-based diet. Research suggests that less than 2 percent of our diet should come from animal foods. In fact, studies have shown that vegetarians get far better nutrition than non-vegetarians. A plant-based diet supplies all vitamins adequately except for vitamin B-12, which can easily be provided in the form of a supplement.

Not only is a plant-based diet nutritionally sound but the people who consume one tend to be healthier and live longer than those who eat animal products on a regular basis. A 12-year study of more than 34,000 Seventh-Day Adventists in California, most of whom were vegetarians, found that on average, group members lived 10 years longer than the general population, and remained healthier and had fewer complaints of illness than non-members.

Converting to a plant-based diet yields many benefits including:

♦ **Longevity:** The World Health Organization (WHO) cites a **low** intake of fruits and vegetables among the top 10 risk factors contributing to death.

♦ **Heart Disease:** According to data from the Health Professionals Follow-Up Study and the Nurses' Health Study, individuals who regularly consume fruits and vegetables significantly reduce their risk of coronary heart disease.

♦ **Stroke:** A recent study published in the journal *Stroke* found a 58 percent reduced risk of stroke among people who consumed vegetables six to seven days per week compared to those who consumed vegetables only two days a week.

♦ **Cancer:** The National Cancer Institute, in its booklet, "Diet, Nutrition & Cancer Prevention: A Guide to Food," reports that 35 percent of all cancer deaths may be attributed to diet alone. Diets rich in animal products increased the risk for certain cancers, while plant foods offer significant protection. Evidence suggests that fruits and vegetables protect against gastrointestinal and smoking related cancers, including cancers of the lung, colon, stomach, mouth, esophagus, bladder and prostate. Evidence also suggests that a diet rich in whole grains can help protect against various cancers, particularly colon, stomach and endometrial.

♦ **Ideal Body Weight:** Because plant foods tend to be much lower in calories and more filling than animal foods, achieving and maintaining an ideal body weight is accomplished with ease by adhering to a plant-based diet.

♦ **Premature Aging:** Plant foods may also help delay the onset of premature aging, while animal foods appear to accelerate the aging process.

♦ **Other:** Plant-based diets have also proven beneficial in the prevention of macular degeneration, diverticulosis (an intestinal disorder) and neural tube defects (a spinal cord defect that can occur in infants when a pregnant women is deficient in folic acid).

Let's be clear: This is not the same thing as adding a few apples and some broccoli into your daily mix of lunch-meats, fast-food and other unhealthy items. It means replacing nearly all of your meals throughout the day, most days of the week, with plant foods. For example, your daily luncheon meat sandwich on white bread made with bleached flour, can be replaced with peanut-butter and jam (no preservatives or additives, low-sugar/low-fat varieties) on whole-grain bread.

The Daily Dozen—Power Up Your Health Today

One of the best ways to power up health is by including the Daily Dozen foods into your daily regimen. The Daily Dozen foods are capable of preventing and/or reversing heart disease, cancer, stroke, diabetes, hypertension, arthritis and premature aging, and in turn, increasing life span. They are in essence, the best of the best.

In Appendix B you will find a helpful menu planner (and Lifestyle Diary) with each of the Daily Dozen foods listed as a way to remind you of the importance of these foods and to help you plan your meals around them. They are indeed "nature's pharmacy" because they all have the power to heal and protect us from disease.

My Daily Dozen foods include:

- Tomatoes
- Spinach
- Broccoli
- Apples
- Whole grains
- Blueberries
- Nuts
- Fatty fish (wild, not farm-raised)
- Green tea
- Pomegranate juice
- Legumes
- Red wine

Tomatoes and Tomato-Based Products

Tomatoes provide a major source of the antioxidant lycopene. Studies have found a reduced risk of cancer and increased cancer survival in individuals who consume high amounts of tomato-based products. One study found that men who consume more than 10 servings per week of tomatoes and tomato products had a 35 percent decreased risk of prostate cancer compared to those who ate less than 1.5 servings a week. European researchers have recently found a significant association between a high dietary intake of lycopene and a 48 percent reduced risk of heart disease.

To increase your intake of lycopene, try a garden salad with fresh sliced tomatoes. Or drink low-sodium V8 juice, or have a bowl of tomato-based soup. Increased consumption of concentrated tomato sauces, stews and soups are encouraged, as they contain up to five times more lycopene than fresh tomatoes.

Spinach

Spinach contains indole-3 carbinol, which inhibits growth of cancer cells in the laboratory. It's packed with iron and folic acid. Folic acid reduces blood levels of homocysteine. Spinach also contains the phytochemicals lutein and zeaxanthin, which offer protection from macular degeneration, a leading cause of blindness. Other green, leafy vegetables such as kale, Swiss chard and collard greens also provide benefits similar to spinach.

Increase your intake of spinach with a garden salad made from fresh baby spinach leaves (or chopped kale, collard or turnip greens), or a serving of steamed spinach with a touch of olive oil, garlic and/or lemon. Use organic baby spinach leaves as a base for your garden salads as opposed to Romaine and other types of lettuce, to insure plenty of this powerful vegetable in your diet.

Broccoli

Broccoli is the king of produce when it comes to basic nutrients. The indole-3 carbinol, as well as sulforaphane, in broccoli, destroy cancer cells in lab experiments. When scientists at the World Cancer Research Fund reviewed more than 200 scientific studies involving humans and animals, they found convincing evidence that increased intake of cruciferous vegetables like broccoli significantly reduced the risk of some cancers. And ounce for ounce, broccoli contains as much calcium as a glass of milk and is a rich source of vitamins A and C. One medium spear of broccoli also contains about three times the amount of fiber as in a slice of whole-grain bread. Other members of the cruciferous family include cabbage, cauliflower, kale and Brussels sprouts. Broccoli *sprouts* contain 10 to 100 times more cancer-fighting compounds than broccoli spears.

Add cuts of broccoli, or the sprouts, to salads. Cuts can be eaten raw, dipped in garlic sauce or other vegetable-dipping sauces. Broccoli can also be steamed.

Apple

According to the latest research, the old saying, "An apple a day keeps the doctor away," is fact, not just folklore. A major review study published in the May 2004 issue of the *Nutrition Journal* provides dozens of reasons to enjoy an apple every day. A review study is one that looks at the results of many other studies. This one included an analysis of 85 studies. Apples were found to be most consistently associated with a reduced risk of heart disease, cancer, asthma and Type 2 diabetes when compared to other fruits and vegetables. Eating apples was also associated with increased lung function and increased weight loss.

Apples are an excellent source of both insoluble and soluble fiber. Soluble fiber can help lower cholesterol levels and reduce your risk of hardening of the arteries, heart attack and stroke. Adding just one large apple to the daily diet has been shown to decrease serum cholesterol 8-11 percent. Eating two large apples a day has lowered cholesterol levels by up to 16 percent!

Researchers in Finland followed over 5,000 Finnish men and women for over 20 years. Those who ate the most apples and other flavonoid-rich (flavonoids give fruits and vegetables their color) foods were found to have a 20 percent lower risk of heart disease than those who ate the least of these foods.

Apples have also been shown to greatly inhibit the growth of liver and colon cancer cells in several studies. In one study, the growth of cancerous cells in the liver was inhibited by 39 percent by extracts of whole Fuji apples and 57 percent by whole Red Delicious extracts.

An apple a day may also offer significant protection against breast cancer, suggests an animal study published in the March 2005 *Journal of Agricultural and Food Chemistry*. When mice with breast cancer were fed the human equivalent of one, three or six apples a day for six months, their tumors shrank by 25 percent, 25 percent and 61 percent, respectively. This study demonstrates that the protective effects of apples are dose-dependent, meaning, the more apples eaten the more the protection.

Out of 10 varieties commonly consumed in the U.S., Fuji and Red Delicious apples have the highest antioxidant activity. Whole apples appear to be far more beneficial than apple juice. Processing apples greatly reduces their antioxidant activity, in some instances by up to 97 percent.

According to the Environmental Working Group's 2003 report, "Shopper's Guide to Pesticides in Produce," apples are among the 12 foods on which pesticide residues have been most frequently found. Therefore, individuals wanting to avoid pesticide-associated health risks should choose organically-grown apples.

Apples' protective effects against free radical damage to cholesterol (oxidation of "bad" cholesterol) reach their peak at three hours following apple consumption and drop off after 24 hours, meaning that they must be consumed daily in order to reap these benefits. Having trouble chewing down apples? Try apple sauce. But read the ingredients. Eat only sauces with just two ingredients: apples, water.

Whole Grains

Whole grains are rich in antioxidants, tumor suppressors, insulin regulators, cholesterol reducers and a broad range of nutrients including B vitamins, vitamins E and K, calcium, iron, magnesium and fiber. Studies indicate that replacing refined grains with whole grains can lower the risk of many chronic diseases including heart disease, stroke, Type 2 diabetes, obesity and even cancer. These benefits are most pronounced for those consuming three servings of whole grains daily, but even as little as one serving daily can offer benefit.

Researchers at the Harvard School of Public Health analyzed diet and health records of over 27,000 men, 40-75, over a period of 14 years, and found that those with the highest whole grain intake (about 40g per day) cut heart disease risk by almost 20 percent—but even those eating just 25 grams daily cut their CHD risk by 15 percent (*American Journal of Clinical Nutrition,* Dec. 2004*).*

A second study published in the *Archives of Internal Medicine* (2004) found a 14 percent reduction in heart disease risk and a 25 percent reduction in dying from heart disease for each 10 grams of fiber consumed daily. In other words, the fiber in whole grains appears to reduce the risk of heart disease, and makes it less serious if it does occur. A high intake of fiber-rich whole grains was also found to reduce the risk of rectal cancer by an impressive 66 percent, according to research published in the *American Journal of Clinical Nutrition* (2004).

If you are concerned about your weight, a diet rich in whole grains can help. Researchers studied the diet and health records of 72,000 men and found that those who ate 40 grams of whole grains per day cut middle-age weight gain by up to 3.5 pounds. Just one cup of cooked oatmeal or two slices of whole-wheat bread would provide this amount of whole grain. (*American Journal of Clinical Nutrition,* 2004*).*

Researchers at Tufts University found that people who eat three or more servings of whole grains a day, especially from high-fiber cereals, are less likely to develop insulin resistance and metabolic syndrome, common precursors of both Type 2 diabetes and cardiovascular disease (*Diabetes Care,* 2004*).*

Examples of whole grains include oat bran (perhaps the healthiest whole grain), oatmeal, barley, whole wheat flour, whole wheat bread, whole wheat pasta and brown rice. Many people make the mistake of believing "wheat bread" or "wheat pasta" is the same as "whole wheat" bread and pasta. For better health, the product should state "whole" wheat or "whole" grain.

Blueberries

Researchers at the USDA Human Nutrition Center (HNRCA) have found that wild blueberries rank #1 in antioxidant activity when compared to 40 other fresh fruits and vegetables. Antioxidants in blueberries (known as anthocyanidins) have the ability to neutralize harmful free radicals that have been linked to heart disease, cancer, stroke, mental deterioration, cataracts and other age-related illnesses and disease. Anthocyanin—the pigment that makes blueberries blue—is thought to be responsible for this major health benefit.

In animal studies, researchers have found that blueberries help protect the brain from oxidative stress and may reduce the effects of age-related conditions such as Alzheimer's disease or dementia. Researchers found that diets rich in blueberries significantly improved both the learning capacity and motor skills of aging rats, making them mentally equivalent with much younger rats.

Blueberries can also help improve learning and memory. Spanish researchers at the University of Barcelona found that after eight weeks of feeding lab rats various blueberries, they saw a reversal of age-related declines in the rats' ability to find their way through the Morris water maze, a measure of the animals' spatial learning ability and memory. Phytonutrients found in blueberries have the ability to cross the blood-brain barrier and affect areas of the brain responsible for learning and memory.

Eating plenty of blueberries may significantly lessen brain damage from strokes and other neurological disorders, suggests a study published in the May 2005 issue of the *Journal of Experimental Neurology*. Rats fed diets enriched with blueberries suffered the loss of much fewer brain cells and recovered significantly more of their ability to move following a stroke. Blueberries may also reduce the buildup of bad cholesterol that contributes to cardiovascular disease and stroke, according to scientists at the University of California at Davis.

In addition to their powerful anthocyanins, blueberries contain another antioxidant compound called *ellagic acid*, which blocks metabolic pathways that can lead to cancer. In a study of 1,271 elderly people in New Jersey, those who ate the most strawberries (another berry that contains ellagic acid) were three times less likely to develop cancer than those who ate few or no strawberries. In addition to containing ellagic acid, blueberries are high in the soluble fiber pectin, which has been shown to lower cholesterol and to prevent bile acid from being transformed into a potentially cancer-causing form.

Laboratory studies published in the September 2005 issue of the *Journal of Agricultural and Food Chemistry* show that phenolic compounds in blueberries can inhibit colon cancer growth and kill existing cancer cells in the body. If fresh blueberries are not available, substitute frozen or dried berries, and even blueberry juice, which is sold in bottles. Other varieties of berries rich in antioxidants include cranberries, blackberries, raspberries and strawberries.

Enjoy blueberries mixed into your favorite cereal, yogurt or as is. If you don't like the taste of straight blueberries, you can eat them in the form of a puree: health-food stores usually sell whole-grain bars filled with blueberry paste; and all-natural scones and muffins with blueberries. Often, these foods are sweetened with cane juice or organic sugar, and these simple carbs are well worth the antioxidant levels in blueberries.

Nuts

According to results from the Physicians' Health Study, consuming nuts two or more times a week can reduce the risk of sudden cardiac death by almost 50 percent and lowers the risk of cardiac death from all causes by 30 percent. Nuts are also rich in vitamin E, and "healthy" fats that improve cholesterol profile. Two of the healthiest varieties of nuts include walnuts and pecans. Walnuts and pecans contain ellagic acid, discussed above.

Add a serving of nuts to your breakfast cereal or salad, or enjoy them in their raw form. Avoid heavily salted nuts. Nuts are also high in calories and can contribute to weight gain, so be careful not to overindulge. One handful daily should be sufficient.

Fatty Fish

Fish such as salmon, tuna and mackerel contain high amounts of the very heart-healthy omega-3 fatty acids. *Choose wild salmon over the farmed variety, and limit consumption of **farmed** salmon to an 8-ounce serving no more than once a month; the contaminants from environmental pollution pose cancer risks to humans. You can find wild salmon at most fish markets and online. Most canned salmon is also of the wild variety. When preparing salmon, trim the skin and visible fat, since contaminants are stored in the fat. Grilling or broiling salmon can also help remove excess fat and toxins.*

Always stick with the wild varieties when it comes to salmon, or smaller less toxic fish such as tilapia, sardines and shrimp. If you choose to eat tuna, chunk-light is your best bet; it's much lower in mercury.

Green Tea

"Tea is one of the single best cancer fighters you can put in your body," states Dr. Mitchell Gaynor, director of medical oncology at the world-renowned Strong Cancer Prevention Center in New York. Green tea has been shown to significantly reduce risk for heart disease, cancer and stroke when consumed frequently. The protective effects of green tea can be attributed to its high concentration of a compound known as EGCG.

EGCG has the ability to kill cancer cells without causing harm to surrounding healthy cells. No prescription drug can make that claim. Numerous scientific studies have provided so much additional evidence on the benefits of drinking green tea, that it's now an acknowledged cancer preventative in Japan.

Green tea can also: limit damage caused by diabetes; protect the liver against damage and viral infections; increase bone density in men and women; benefit people with rheumatoid arthritis; and act as a weight-loss aid.

Most research indicates that the disease-preventative effects of green tea occur at levels of about 5-10 cups daily. I highly recommend a daily green tea extract supplement in addition to enjoying a few cups of freshly brewed tea.

Although green and black teas come from the same plant, green tea leaves are steamed and dried rather than fermented, thus preserving more antioxidants. An analysis of 20 common tea brands found the highest antioxidant content in Celestial Seasonings Green Tea, Lipton Green Tea, and Bigelow Darjeeling Blend after three minutes of brewing time.

Pomegranate Juice

Enjoying a daily 8-ounce glass of pomegranate juice may be one of the most important steps you can take to protect yourself against cardiovascular disease and certain cancers. Pomegranate juice is a rich source of flavonoids, potent antioxidants. One glass contains more antioxidants than green tea. Mice injected with human prostate cancer cells and fed pomegranate extract experienced a significantly inhibited growth of tumors and an increased survival rate.

One glass of pure pomegranate juice per day is all that's required for better health. If you are diabetic or suffer from hypoglycemia, you may want to consume small amounts throughout the day to limit abnormal spikes in blood sugar.

Legumes

Legumes are often called "the poor people's meat." However, they might be better known as the "healthy people's meat." Common legumes include black, kidney, lima, navy and pinto beans. Diets rich in legumes have been shown to lower cholesterol levels, improve blood glucose control in diabetics, and reduce the risk of numerous cancers.

Legumes contain many important nutrients and phytochemicals, and when combined with grains, they form a complete protein. According to studies conducted by the United States Department of Agriculture, richly colored dried beans offer a high degree of antioxidant protection. In fact, small red kidney beans rated the highest just ahead of blueberries.

Legumes are an excellent low-fat source of protein, complex carbohydrates and fiber and are rich in folic acid, molybdenum, phosphorus, iron, magnesium, manganese and potassium. Folic acid and B-6 help lower levels of the amino acid homocysteine.

Legumes also contain an abundance of fiber, and as a result, have the ability to lower cholesterol and improve cardiovascular health.

Beans also contain significant amounts of antioxidants that provide additional protection against the development of cardiovascular disease and cancer as well as other illnesses linked to free radical damage. Researchers with the United States Department of Agriculture analyzed antioxidant levels in over 100 different foods. The red kidney, pinto and black varieties were all ranked near the top of this list with respect to their antioxidant content.

As noted above, legumes are also protective against cancer. In one analysis of dietary data collected by validated food frequency questionnaires in 1991 and 1995, from 90,630 women in the Nurses Health Study II, researchers found a significantly reduced frequency of breast cancer in those women who consumed a higher intake of common beans or lentils. Eating beans or lentils two or more times per week was associated with a 24 percent reduced risk of breast cancer. The high fiber content of most beans prevents blood sugar levels from rising too rapidly after a meal, making these beans an especially good choice for individuals with diabetes, insulin resistance or hypoglycemia.

You can enjoy beans in soups, salads or just by themselves.

Red Wine

Red wine, when consumed in moderation, appears to reduce risk of heart disease and may help extend life. A recent study published in the May 2006 issue of the *New England Journal of Medicine* found a 41 percent lower risk of heart disease in men with moderate alcohol intakes (1-2 drinks daily) compared to those who abstained from alcohol. Only a 7 percent reduction in heart disease risk was seen in men who enjoyed a drink once weekly.

One drink is defined as 12 ounces of beer, **4 ounces of wine** or 1 ounce of 100-proof whiskey. A second study published in the *Journal of the American Medical Association* found a 32 percent reduction in the risk of death following a heart attack in patients who consumed seven red wine drinks a week in the year prior to their heart attack, compared to those who abstained from drinking.

Other benefits of red wine:

■   Reduces risk of prostate cancer by 50 percent

- Lowers likelihood of blood clots
- Reduces blood pressure
- Lowers risk of Type 2 diabetes
- Fights premature aging
- Recent research suggests that moderate consumption of red wine can also help protect against lung cancer.

Whenever possible, choose red wine over white wine or other types of alcohol (lower antioxidant level). Red wine is rich in resveratrol—a natural antioxidant. For years, researchers have studied resveratrol, linking it to reduced risk of cancer, atherosclerosis, heart disease and brain diseases such as Alzheimer's—all illnesses that are more prevalent as we age.

There is sufficient evidence indicating that calorie restriction can extend life span across a range of species. Studies are now finding that resveratrol may be able to replicate this process, allowing cells to live longer. After screening thousands of molecules, researchers have found that resveratrol mimics calorie restriction in yeast—activating enzymes that slow aging, increasing the stability of DNA, hence extending life span by as much as 70 percent. Researchers suspect plants make these age-slowing molecules as a defense response. Resveratrol may also be of benefit in the prevention of certain cancers and age-related brain disorders.

Just because limited red wine consumption is healthy doesn't mean that it's okay to go out and drink up a storm. For those who choose to drink, the American Heart Association recommends no more than one to two drinks per day for men, and one drink per day for women (because women in general have less muscle and bone than men, and a slower metabolism).

Getting the Most from the Daily Dozen Foods

Sample menu for one day

Breakfast

Bowl of oatmeal mixed with blueberries and/or nuts

4 egg whites (seasoned with "power" spices such as oregano, garlic and parsley)
Pomegranate juice
Green tea

Mid-Morning Snack

Apple or celery w/peanut butter

Lunch

Salad of fresh spinach leaves, broccoli, nuts and tomatoes with extra virgin olive oil and vinegar as dressing

Mid-Afternoon Snack

Whey protein shake with non-fat milk or water (be sure the shake mix isn't artificially sweetened and doesn't contain "artificial flavor." You can find natural shake mixes at a whole-foods or health food store.)

Dinner

6-ounce portion of wild salmon or grilled free-range chicken breast
2 servings of fresh vegetables
Slice of whole grain bread dipped in olive oil with crushed garlic
Glass of red wine

Early Evening Snack

4 ounces of dark chocolate
Green tea

No Need to Ever Count Calories

I have provided a Lifestyle Diary in Appendix B of this book to help you monitor your progress and plan your meals. Instead of providing you with a specific meal plan to follow, which does not take into account your individual preferences, I offer several options from which to choose for breakfast, lunch, dinner and snacks. Remember, since most plant foods are naturally low in calories, you don't need to count calories or measure portions. You will also find an actual sample of my seven-day eating plan in the completed diaries to get a better idea of how to combine certain foods and make healthier selections when it comes to meals.

Other Healthy Plant Foods (Secondary Foods)

Sweet Potatoes

In 1992, the Center for Science in the Public Interest compared the nutritional value of sweet potatoes to all other vegetables. Considering fiber content, complex carbohydrates, protein, vitamins A and C, iron and calcium, the sweet potato ranked highest in nutritional value. According to these criteria, sweet potatoes earned 184 points, 100 points over the next on the list, the white potato. Diabetics and others wanting to avoid glucose highs and lows can safely consume sweet potatoes, which have a low glycemic index. They are also rich in antioxidants, fiber and potassium.

Avocado

Eating as little as half an avocado daily for three weeks improved blood cholesterol in middle-aged women more than a high-complex-carbohydrate diet, according to a study published in the *American Journal of Clinical Nutrition*. The avocado diet reduced total cholesterol by a total of 8 percent.

Enjoy freshly sliced chilled avocado, or as a dip (guacamole) with some baked or whole-grain chips.

Peanut Butter

Peanut butter provides an excellent source of healthy fatty acids, magnesium, folate, vitamin E and fiber. It's also an excellent source of choline, a nutrient required by your brain to stay energetic and alert.

A tablespoon of peanut butter ranges from 90 to 190 calories, so limit daily intake accordingly if you are trying to lose weight.

Yogurt

Probiotics (commonly referred to as "friendly" bacteria) are living microorganisms found in food that are crucial to digestive system health. The integrity of the gut largely relies on the balance between good and bad bacteria. Probiotics help bring balance to the digestive system. Research has shown that adding probiotics to your diet can help improve health of the good bacteria living in the gut, and may help protect both the intestinal lining and the immune system. When taken in conjunction with fiber, probiotics help create anti-cancer compounds.

One of the best food sources of probiotics is yogurt. To get the most health benefits from yogurt, look for the "Live and Active Cultures" seal on the label. L. acidophilus is by far the most commonly added probiotic. Be sure to choose non-or low-fat varieties of plain yogurt, as most flavored yogurts contain unhealthy amounts of sugar and calories. Add fresh blueberries or cinnamon to naturally flavor yogurt and to supercharge the antioxidant content.

Spices

A study of cooking herbs from the U.S. Department of Agriculture (USDA) found that most spices had greater antioxidant power per gram than various fruits and vegetables. Spices contain substances that inhibit cancer-causing enzymes and tumor-stimulating hormones, and slow the lifecycle of cancer cells or encourage their destruction.

Some of the most promising research has been conducted on the herbs turmeric, cinnamon, oregano and sage. One USDA study found that consuming under half a teaspoon daily of cinnamon for 40 days reduced blood levels of sugar and triglycerides by about 25 percent, and cut LDL cholesterol levels by nearly 20 percent.

Use spices generously when cooking for greatest benefit. For a double heap of antioxidant power, sprinkle cinnamon on apple slices.

Dark Chocolate and Cocoa Products

Emerging research has found that dark chocolate and cocoa products may help reduce the risk of cardiovascular disease and diabetes. Dark chocolate and cocoa products are rich in flavonoids, which act as natural antioxidants. Flavonoids help limit arterial damage caused by free radicals. Flavonoids also reduce the ability of platelets in the blood to clot, thus lowering risk for heart attack and stroke. Other studies have indicated that cocoa flavonoids help relax blood vessels by blocking an enzyme that causes inflammation.

Harvard researchers tracked nearly 8,000 males, with an average age of 65. Those men who enjoyed chocolate lived almost a year longer than those who did not.

Chocolate may be endowed with more than just antioxidants. Research published in the *American Journal of Clinical Nutrition* in 1997 showed that one of the fats in chocolate, called stearic acid, can boost HDL levels. Also, when people ate milk chocolate regularly, their levels of LDL didn't increase as might have been expected from fat consumption. Another study found that just 3.5 ounces of dark chocolate lowered blood pressure in a group of men and women after only 15 days.

A few ounces a day of plain dark chocolate are all that's required for better health. The more processed the chocolate is, such as chocolate donuts or "cupcakes" that come in a box, the weaker the level of antioxidants. Avoid dark chocolate candy bars; most contain only a coating of dark chocolate and are filled with unhealthy saturated fat.

Remember: Commercially-made cupcakes, donuts, cookies and ice cream products do not fall under the category of "plain, pure, all-natural dark chocolate." You can find chunks of pure dark chocolate, with varying degrees of sugar content, at most health food stores. Chocolate without added sugar is extremely unpalatable. Milk chocolate has about half the antioxidant punch as dark chocolate.

What About Soy?

Most of the soy grown in the U.S. is used for livestock feed. What is left over is then used for human consumption, mostly in a very processed form, such as soy protein powder, soy protein bars, soy dairy products, soy "burgers" and even soy "chips."

The soy health-hype is driven by population studies showing that people in Asia, who consume much more soy than do Americans, have lower incident rates of certain cancers. This is an associative link between soy consumption and cancer rate; no causal association has been established. There are a few loopholes in these population studies.

First, other variables that may affect cancer rate need to be considered. People in Asia drink far more green tea than U.S. residents. Perhaps this is why some cancer rates are lower in the Far East. Asians also typically eat more vegetables and less fast-food than Americans. Certainly, this affects immunity to disease.

Secondly, the soy that Asians eat is almost always in whole form, such as tofu, tamari and miso. When soy is processed, this changes its molecular makeup, and many whole-soy advocates believe that this change causes a disruption in the way soy's phytoestrogens work inside the human body.

The soy industry's marketing campaign has been brilliant. But many experts are now beginning to catch on to what very well may be the truth about processed soy products. Recent clinical studies have failed to show a protective benefit of soy protein in the diet. Members of the American Heart Association (AHA) nutrition committee reviewed 22 such studies and concluded that eating soy-based foods has only minimal impact on cholesterol and other heart-disease risk factors. The studies indicated that people who ate about 50 grams of soy protein a day reduced LDL (bad) cholesterol by only about 3 percent. Fifty grams of soy a day is a lot. One soy protein bar—or one scoop of soy protein powder—may contain only 15 grams of soy.

Eating large amounts of soy had no effect on other risk factors such as triglycerides or HDL "good" cholesterol. Isoflavones, the key components of soy that make them so potent as a possible substitute for hormone replacement therapy, mean that soy products, while touted as foods and nutritional products—often are used like a hormonal drug.

If you have a diagnosed or undiagnosed thyroid problem, or a history of autoimmune disease, over-consumption of soy isoflavones can potentially trigger a thyroid condition. Soy foods can worsen an existing diagnosed thyroid problem in many people. A recent study (*Journal of Clinical Endocrinology and Metabolism*, 2002) found that millions of Americans have an undiagnosed thyroid condition. The vast majority of thyroid patients are women over 40. This is the same group turning to soy foods in vast numbers.

America's leading alternative doctor, Dr. Andrew Weil, has said this about soy:

"*...you're unlikely to get too many isoflavones as a result of adding soy foods to your diet—but you probably will take in too much if you take soy supplements in pill form. At this point, I can only recommend that you avoid soy supplements entirely.*"

Reduce Your Consumption of Animal Products

During a lifetime, the average meat eater will consume approximately 36 pigs, 36 sheep, 750 chickens and poultry, and seven cows—which translates to 4,200 pounds of beef. Animal products, including cheese, milk and eggs, play a very limited role in a healthful diet. The exception is low-fat organic yogurt with probiotics.

Animal products contain high amounts of saturated fat and cholesterol. Many people worry that removing meat from their diets will eliminate essential proteins and nutrients not found in plant foods. The truth is that meat contains absolutely nothing that you can't get from plant foods (with the exception of vitamin B-12).

When you consume animal products, you also ingest the hormones, drugs and other chemicals given to the animal prior to its slaughter. A diet high in animal products is also associated in one way or another with cancer, stroke, diabetes, arthritis, constipation, obesity, gout, gallstones and kidney stones.

The Adventist Health Study found that men who consumed beef four or more times per week were twice as likely to die from heart disease as men not consuming beef. The World Cancer Research Fund's landmark report, "Food, Nutrition, and the Prevention of Cancer," concluded: "Diets containing substantial amounts of red meat probably increase the risk of colorectal cancer, and such diets possibly increase the risk of pancreatic, breast, prostate, and renal cancers." The organization recommends that red meat, if eaten at all, should be limited to three ounces daily.

Recent findings presented at the 96th Annual Meeting of the American Association for Cancer Research 2005 found that people who ate more than 2 ounces of red meat or pork a day had a 50 percent increased risk of pancreatic cancer.

Completely eliminating all animal products is unrealistic for most people. But you can work on cutting back on animal products, such as giving up the breakfast meats (bacon, ham, sausage) or avoiding fast-food establishments. If you plan on eating dairy products, opt for no-fat or low-fat varieties.

If you continue to consume red meat, always choose the leanest cuts of beef possible. Purchase organic, grass-fed beef and pork and free-range chicken and turkey. Organic, grass-fed cattle are lower in fat, hormones, antibiotics and residue from pesticides, insecticides and herbicides commonly found in grain-fed cattle. Remember, these products may be "healthier" than their conven-

tional counterparts, but they are still considered animal products and as such, their consumption should be limited.

Pay attention to the temperature at which you prepare beef. Cooking at high temperatures increases the production of compounds in meat known as heterocyclic amines. These cause changes in DNA and increase cancer risk. In fact, people who consume meat that is fried or well-done have a greater risk for cancer than those who consume meat cooked in other ways. Always choose rare-to-medium temperatures when preparing red meat.

Increase Intake of Dietary Fiber

Dietary fiber helps reduce heart disease risk and may also help cut risk of some cancers. The Physicians' Health Study found that fewer heart attacks occurred in those who ate more fiber, particularly the soluble type. Because fiber increases the rate at which waste products are removed from the colon and rectum, it also helps reduce exposure to toxic substances produced in the bowel. Estimates indicate that the risk of colorectal cancer in the U.S. could be reduced by as much as 31 percent if Americans increased their fiber intake by an average of 13 grams per day.

The National Cancer Institute suggests a daily intake of 20-35 grams. Increasing your intake of fruits and vegetables, nuts and seeds, legumes, oats and barley can help ensure an optimal level of fiber. If you find it hard to consume enough fiber from diet alone, then a fiber supplement is a good option. Be sure that it contains a mixture of both soluble and insoluble fiber, and is free of added sugars.

Reduce Consumption of the White Death

The average American consumes about 20 teaspoons of refined sugar every day and over 150 lbs of added sugars each year, according to the Center for Science in Public Interest. Sweetened soft drinks, sweetened fruit juices, breakfast cereals and snack foods are major contributors to dietary sugar. Even some *soups* contain sugar, and that is mm, mm, bad!

The term "sugar" includes: corn syrup, molasses, maltodexterin and any word ending in "ose," such as lactose and fructose. The Synergy Eating Plan widens the term "sugar" to include all refined carbohydrates such as white rice, white bread, enriched flours, sugary cereals and pasta made from white flour.

Refined carbohydrates have no place in a healthful diet. All of the vitamins and minerals have been removed from refined carbs, allowing these carbohydrates to be digested and absorbed into the bloodstream very quickly. Each time you consume sugar, insulin levels in your blood increase. Insulin removes sugar from the blood and transports it to the cells where it is stored as fat. Chronically elevated insulin levels can lead to a condition known as insulin resistance, a precursor to Type 2 diabetes, and linked to cardiovascular disease and cancer. High sugar consumption can also lead to weak bones, digestive problems and migraine headaches.

The amount of sugar in just two cans of soda can reduce the efficiency of white blood cells by 92 percent, an effect that can last up to five hours, according to nutritional and environmental expert Kenneth Bock, M.D., Co-Founder and Co-Director of the Rhinebeck Health Center in Rhinebeck, New York. Because white blood cells are essential to a healthy immune system, if you happen to come into contact with a virus or bacteria a few hours after consuming a sweetened drink, your immune system may be unable to fight off the invader.

Guidelines for reducing sugar intake

- Don't be fooled by those commercials showing "moms" serving their kids some brightly colored drink that's high in vitamin C. Manufacturers market these beverages as great sources of vitamin C when, in reality, they are nothing more than fruit-flavored sugar water.
- Beware of specialty coffee drinks. They can be a significant source of sugar.
- Replace sugary breakfast cereals with whole grain cereals that are lower in sugars (read the labels).

When Fat is Healthy

Much of the research involving dietary fat indicates that the type and ratio of fats in the diet have more of an influence on health than does the amount of total fat. There is an abundance of scientific evidence documenting the health risks associated with an excess consumption of polyunsaturated fats.

The two major categories of polyunsaturated fats are omega-3 and omega-6 essential fatty acids. Most Americans consume excessive amounts of omega-6 fatty acids (from vegetable oils) and not nearly enough omega-3s. A proper balance of omega-3s and omega-6s is required for optimal health. The ideal ratio of omega-6 to omega-3 fats is 2:1. The average American's ratio of omega-6 to omega-3 is closer to 10:1. This imbalance can increase risk for an assortment of medical conditions including stroke.

In order to properly balance this ratio, you must increase intake of omega-3s while decreasing intake of omega-6s. This is best accomplished by avoiding or limiting intake of foods rich in omega-6 oils such as fried foods, processed foods, baked goods and certain vegetable oils, while upping intake of omega-3s. (You can gain even more benefit by replacing oils high in omega-6s with those rich in a third type of fatty acid known as omega-9, such as extra virgin olive oil.)

Although salmon and other fatty fish are rich sources of omega-3 fatty acids, most fish found in our markets and restaurants contain dangerously high levels of mercury and PCBs (See Chapter 6). Other food sources for omega-3s are ground flaxseeds, and walnuts. However, the best source for omega-3s are fish oil supplements, 2-4 grams daily.

Eating Less Doubles Life Span of Lab Animals

Eat less for a longer and livelier life span. Caloric restriction (CR) is currently the only intervention proven to increase life span in lab animals.

In studies involving rodents and lower primates, CR has been found to extend life and to reduce the occurrence of disease later in life. In animal studies, CR delayed age-related processes. In a study with monkeys—in which one was fed amply—and one was on CR, by the time they reached middle-aged years (in monkey terms), the monkey fed "normally" was already showing signs of age and lethargy, plus early heart disease. The monkey on CR was still spry and energetic, with no signs of heart disease. In fact, of the 300 known biomarkers of aging, 90 percent of them indicate that animals put on a calorie-restricted diet stay younger.

Researchers have observed the following benefits with CR:

- Significant increase in life span
- Can reduce diabetes risk

- Improves cholesterol profile
- Improves immune system function
- Lowers blood pressure
- Helps keep fat away from abdomen
- Reduces damage to DNA and slowed progression of cancerous tumors
- Reduction in free radical damage

According to some researchers in the field of aging and longevity, CR in humans could increase the average life span of 75 years by 30 years if current research holds true in human trials.

Individuals who have experimented with short-term CR (less than two years) commonly report better health and increased vitality. In the first scientifically controlled trial of CR in humans, known as Biosphere 2, four men and four women were sealed inside a closed ecological system for two years and put on a low-calorie diet that was for the most part plant-based. During that time, the male subjects lost an average of 18 percent of their total body weight; women, 10 percent. Blood pressure decreased an average of 20 in all subjects, and diabetic indicators were all reduced by almost 30 percent. Cholesterol levels were also reduced more than 35 percent.

Although it may sound severe, in actuality, CR does not imply starvation or constant hunger pangs. It simply translates to making sensible choices when it comes to meals. Rodents and other animals put on CR were fed 30-50 percent fewer calories than what they were normally accustomed to eating. Switching from the typical American diet to the Synergy Eating Plan will automatically reduce your overall caloric intake by up to 50 percent, leave you with a feeling of satiety throughout the day, and provide lasting health and wellness benefits.

"But I hardly eat, and I'm still fat. Isn't this caloric restriction?" It isn't just the total daily calories that make a difference. It's what you eat, how often, and when. People who claim they "hardly eat" and are still overweight, have several things in common. They eat only once or twice a day. Their diet lacks nutrients. They don't exercise; or if they do, it is of poor quality.

If you go long stretches without food, even if your total intake is low in calories, these long periods of "famine" will trick your body into reacting as though there really is a famine: It will hold on to stored fat, making it difficult or impossible to lose weight.

CR works when the total calories are spread throughout the day, when the person grazes from morning till evening. Overweight people who "hardly eat" almost always skip breakfast and lunch. This really slows metabolism. And when they do eat, it's not usually a lot of fruits and vegetables. Thus, much of their meager supply of calories is "empty" calories.

Consume Smaller Meals More Often

If you dream of fitting into that elegant dress on display in the store window, or looking good on the beach, then eating four to six smaller meals and snacks each day is the only way to go.

Optimal health and longevity not only depend on eating certain types of foods, but the timing and portions of your meals as well. Skipping meals does not help you lose weight and can adversely affect your health. People who eat smaller, more frequent meals have consistently lower cholesterol levels than people who consume larger meals less often.

Some people skip meals to lose weight. But people who eat breakfast are less likely to be overweight, and morning meals also may help maintain weight loss. Although it seems counter-intuitive, eating more often—not less often—actually helps control weight. Studies have demonstrated that those who eat four to six smaller meals per day have less body fat than those consuming two or three meals daily, despite the fact that both groups take in about the same amount of calories.

Eating increases your metabolic rate (the rate at which you burn calories) because it takes energy to break down and digest food. As mentioned prior, consuming only one or two meals a day actually fools your body into thinking that it's in a state of starvation, and thus, metabolism slows. You can crank it up by eating several smaller meals more frequently. Because your body's metabolic rate has a natural cycle of highs and lows, peaking late in the day and dropping to its lowest point during sleep, you should avoid large meals late at night, especially right before bedtime.

Eating one or two larger meals rather than five or six smaller meals and snacks throughout the day can also impact energy levels. Consuming a big meal can cause your blood sugar levels to fall and lead to fatigue and sleepiness. Think about how many times you have been overcome with extreme sleepiness shortly after eating a generous meal. Spacing out smaller meals and snacks throughout the day helps your body avoid dramatic fluctuations in blood sugar and improves energy levels and performance.

For some, switching to smaller, more frequent meals is relatively easy. For others, it can be a hassle. Bear in mind that you don't have to actually consume four, five or six entire meals every few hours; you just have to eat something healthful such as a serving of fruit or a handful of nuts. The best way to accomplish this is to eat three normal, but smaller meals with snacks in between. Once you regularly eat this way, you will begin to notice the benefits, including a satisfied feeling throughout the day and greater success with portion control. Your energy level will be even and you will avoid those late afternoon slumps.

Drink More Clean Water

Your body consists of approximately 70 percent water. So vital is water to survival that you could not function more than a few days without it. By contrast, you could survive up to six weeks without food.

Supplying your body with plenty of fresh, clean water each day is essential for optimal health and functioning. The quality of the water we drink is just as important as the quantity. Long-term consumption of unfiltered tap water, which is loaded with harmful impurities (See Chapter 6), can have damaging effects on your health.

Because most of us do not have access to pure glacier water, our next best choice becomes purified tap or bottled water. About 25 percent of the bottled waters consumed in the U.S. come from municipal water supplies and are treated extensively to remove many of the contaminants that are harmful to your health.

Many authorities recommend drinking approximately 1/2 ounce of water per pound of body weight. This means that a 140 lb individual would require about 70 ounces, or about nine cups of water per day. If you are active, the recommendation is even higher. A simple means for assessing your hydration status is by checking the color of your urine. Very light to clear-colored urine indicates that you are likely well-hydrated. Dark urine can be an indication of dehydration and a signal to drink more water. I recommend sipping on water through the day. Also keep in mind that many beverages such as coffee, tea and juice contain water that counts towards your daily consumption.

In a Nutshell

You really are what you eat, and what you eat and drink can have a profound impact on your current state of health and the total number of years you'll live. For health and longevity, you must not only take precautions to avoid foods that have been deemed unhealthy, but just as important, you must increase your intake of those which have been shown to protect against illness and disease.

Simply put, eliminate or significantly reduce your consumption of animal products, refined carbohydrates, processed and convenience foods, sugar, artificial sweeteners/preservatives and hydrogenated vegetable oils, while increasing your intake of plant foods.

A simple rule of thumb to follow is: *"The closer to nature a food is, the better it likely is for you."*

In this chapter, I've provide you with specific foods and techniques that have been proven to improve health and increase life span. Research suggests that such an eating plan can add 10-15 years to your life, not to mention improve the way you look and feel. Best of all, my eating plan is simple to follow (assuming you have the will to follow it). It does not involve counting calories or points, measuring portions or eliminating a specific food group. To help you track your dietary habits (and lifestyle habits), I have created the Lifestyle Diary which can be found at the back of this book or which can be downloaded @ www.BrandywineChiropractic.com.

I recommend you begin your new eating plan today by first going through your refrigerator and cabinets and ridding yourself of all unhealthy food items. These may include processed and convenience foods, all foods containing hydrogenated oils, baked goods, convenience foods and those high in sugar. Your body will indeed thank you for it!

Next, head to the market or your local health food store and stock up on the antioxidant-rich fruits and vegetables, whole grains and healthy beverages mentioned throughout this chapter. As you consume healthy foods and beverages, visualize your body sailing closer towards optimal health and further away from illness and disease. At all times, you should view your body as a finely tuned engine. Feed it good and it will run well for a very long time. Feed it poorly and you'll be spending plenty of time for repairs at doctors' offices and hospitals.

Chapter 4 Goals:

✓ Eliminate or significantly reduce your consumption of animal products, refined carbohydrates, processed and convenience foods, sugar, artificial sweeteners and preservatives, hydrogenated oils, trans fatty acids and unfiltered tap water.

✓ Adopt a plant-based diet that is rich in organic fruits and vegetables, nuts and seeds, legumes, healthy oils and wild varieties of fish.

✓ Increase your daily intake of the Daily Dozen foods for improved protection against illness and disease.

✓ Consume smaller more frequent meals/snack each day to help stabilize blood sugar levels, improve metabolism and control appetite.

✓ As you consume healthy foods and beverages, visualize your body moving closer towards optimal health and further away from illness and disease.

Chapter 5

Exercise—How Much Do You Really Need?

Life Extension Value: 1-2 Years

"Those who think they have no time for bodily exercise will sooner or later have to find time for illness." ~Edward Stanley

Research suggests that exercise plays a huge role in keeping the body and mind in top shape *well into the eighth and ninth decade of life.* Unfortunately our nation is very lazy as a whole, with only 40 percent of Americans exercising frequently enough to yield health benefits. What's the remaining more-than-half the U.S. population thinking? That luck and wishful thinking alone will keep them healthy and active well into their 80s? Even something as fundamental and as simple as walking can make a difference. If the entire U.S. inactive population would just turn off the TV and walk only one hour every day, five days a week, then the costs of annual medical care and lost productivity from heart disease could be slashed by $4 billion, according to the *Archives of Family Medicine.*

But once again, it's important to drill in the hardcore facts: "Walking an hour a day" does not include any walking you do on the job that you think adds up to one hour by the time your shift is over. It does not include any walking you do around the house that may add up to 60 minutes by bedtime. Unless you have wings, you have no choice but to walk every day somewhere, and of course if you clicked a stopwatch every time you got up and moved, by nightfall you'd probably have 60 minutes on the stopwatch. But with so many people overweight, and so many people sick, the walking we normally do in everyday life obviously isn't cutting it.

In fact, a lot of people will do all it takes to get out of walking. Sadly, many men and women have convinced their doctors that walking is bad for them, and hence, their doctors have issued them handicap permits for their vehicles. This way, they get to park as close to the store's entrance as possible. Some handicaps are "invisible," such as peripheral vascular disease (PVD), in that the person may appear "normal." If someone with PVD is walking, chances are pretty high that the discomfort will be evident—either in the patient's face, or gait.

But if you observe enough people exiting their vehicles in the handicap spots, quite a few of them don't seem the least bit in pain or discomfort as they head toward their destination; some will even walk up a few steps leading to the entrance doors without any problem. How painful is walking, when that person appears to be very comfortable as he or she walks toward their destination? It's difficult to look comfortable and walk smoothly, when walking is painful. A medical condition doesn't mean a person shouldn't walk more than 50 yards. In fact, some medical conditions evolve (either wholly or in part) because the person never walked enough in the first place!

For example, neuropathy is a complication of diabetes. Exercise is one of the best things a diabetic can do to manage the disease. Neuropathy makes walking hurt. But doctors recommend that people with neuropathy walk to help manage the condition and lessen the pain! And guess what doctors vehemently recommend to their patients with PVD: Walk! Some people with handicap permits are obese, and use that as the excuse for the permit. I once knew a 380-pound, 20-something woman whose only condition was the 380 pounds. She had a permit. Nobody doubts that a lot of excess fat on the body can make walking uncomfortable, especially on the back and knees. But the solution is to walk *more*, not less! The more this woman, and others like her, avoid walking, the more they'll ultimately suffer. In short, many people use the existence of a medical condition, or the inability to run, as an excuse for acquiring handicap parking permits, so that they don't have to walk much.

Check out escalators at airports or shopping malls—compare the number of people on them, to the number walking up the steps beside the escalators. Observe the hoards of people on those moving conveyors that link buildings together, compared to the people walking on the regular floors. Get a load of the people who take elevators just to go up—or down—a few flights! Look at how slowly most people walk—not while they are examining price tags at a shopping center—but while they are walking across a parking lot; they literally poke along! Yes, we are a pathetically lazy nation indeed!

Exercise and Life Expectancy

Being in prime shape is essential for increasing life expectancy. People who keep their body fit tend to live longer than those who do not. Being fit is also a better predictor of potential life span than other variables, such as smoking, high blood pressure, heart problems, high cholesterol and diabetes.

A review of 44 papers revealed that the more physical activity a person did, the lower the death rate from all causes of death. It has been shown that as you increase the number of calories burned up with exercise from 500 to 3,500, your chance of dying goes down, and you live longer. In a study of 17,000 Harvard alumni men, the more calories that were burned up by exercise in a week, the lower the risk of death.

Studies have shown that death rates can be 25 percent-33 percent lower among people who use 2,000 or more calories during exercise per week. Burning up 3,500 calories a week has been shown to lower death rates by up to 50 percent. This can amount to an increase of 1—2 years of life expectancy!

Benefits of Regular Exercise

Moderate physical activity just 30 minutes a day 3-5 days per week can significantly improve your overall health, well-being and quality of life. The following benefits of exercise can be achieved by virtually everyone, regardless of age, sex, race or physical ability.

- Reduces your risk of heart disease, stroke, high blood pressure, osteoporosis, diabetes and obesity.
- Reduces your risk for cancers of the colon, prostate, uterus, and breast.
- Increases your life expectancy by 1—2 years.
- Keeps joints, tendons and ligaments flexible so it's easier to move around.
- Reduces many of the effects of aging.
- Boosts the activity of the immune system.
- Contributes to your mental well-being and helps treat depression.

- Helps relieve stress and anxiety.
- Increases your energy and endurance
- Helps deepen shut-eye and cut the time it takes to fall asleep.
- Reduces the urge for a cigarette for those trying to quit.
- Significantly improves mental skills that decline with age.
- Helps maintain or revitalize performance and satisfaction in the bedroom.
- Helps you maintain a normal weight by increasing your metabolism (the rate you burn calories).

Exercise is the most simple and effective way to advance your chances of longevity and reduce the likelihood of impairment. Is it a coincidence that fitness guru Jack LaLanne is still going strong in his 90s? And contrary to popular belief, he does **not** exercise eight hours a day. He's a businessman eight hours a day. But the time he does spend exercising is spent very wisely.

Even if exercise had no impact on life span, would you rather spend the last 15 years of your life with aches, pains and a shuffling gait? Or would you rather be comfortably moving with a perk right up to your last days? When you visit a department store during your golden years, will you be asking an employee where the canes are? Or where the tennis rackets are? Ever see those ads in catalogues for decorative canes? They're becoming hot these days. But a flashy, sparkly cane— when in use by a senior citizen—is no match for an old tennis racket— when in use by a senior citizen, in terms of making someone look cool.

"Okay, then just how much exercise do I really need to fire up my health?"

Exercise need not be strenuous to bring about many health benefits. How *long* you exercise may be more important than how *hard or intensely* you exercise when it comes to cardio health. Thirty minutes of brisk exercise five to six days per week is all it takes to achieve the health benefits associated with exercise. Exercise can "teach" your body to remain youthful well into old age. Much of the deterioration attributed to aging is linked to physical inactivity. Exercise can "teach" your body to remain youthful well into old age. Most would agree that it's not so bad living to the age of 100 if you feel like you're only 70 or 80.

Why Haven't YOU Been Exercising?

"I'm too old! What good will it do me NOW?"

We can't stop time from marching ahead and dragging us with it. However, an accumulating body of evidence has shown that we can alter the rate at which our bodies progress through our lifecycle. It's possible for many of us to be in better condition in our 70s than we were in our 40s and 50s…if we just make time for consistent exercise.

Recent studies indicate that between the ages of 30 and 70, many of the symptoms and conditions that were traditionally associated with normal aging are in fact the result of sedentary lifestyles. Studies have shown that regular exercise by middle-aged and elderly people can set back the clock 20-40 years when compared to those who do little or no exercise. Test results show that no matter when a person starts to exercise, significant improvement can be achieved. One of the groups tested had an average age of 90.

Older people can achieve the same percentage gains in performance as the young, according to Dr. H.A. deVries, past director of the Andrus Gerontology Center at the University of Southern California, and a respected pioneer in the field. In one study of more than 200 men and women 56 to 87, "dramatic changes" were observed after just six weeks of exercising three to five times a week. Study participants became as fit and energetic as people 20 to 30 years younger!

Dr. Everett L. Smith, director of the Biogerontology Laboratory at the University of Wisconsin, has shown that among once sedentary women in their 50s who participated in an aerobic dance program for six years, fitness improved by 23 percent and they experienced **none** of the functional declines typically seen with increasing age! This group appears to have stopped the clock at an age when functional declines are usually apparent. Dr. Smith also compared bone loss among women in their 80s. With those women who did seated exercises for 30 minutes, three times a week for three years, bone mineral density actually **increased** by 2.29 percent, whereas in a similar group of inactive women, bone **loss** averaged 3.28 percent.

"But I have no time to exercise!"

The concept of "time constraints" is all in most peoples' heads. If you were paid $100 to exercise one hour a day, you'd have no problem finding that hour. The issue is priority. As the saying goes, "Excuses are the nails used to build a house of failure." Many people work 10-12 hours a day, come home to several hungry and needy kids, and still find time to honor their body with exercise, be it 20 minutes first thing in the morning before the kids get up, during work lunch breaks (a 20-minute brisk outdoor walk will recharge you far more than a 20-minute "power nap" at your desk that will only leave you feeling groggy when you awaken), or barricading themselves in their bedroom for 30 minutes right after work. Hang a "Do Not Disturb" sign on your door if you must. If you do not make time for better health now, you will surely have to make time for illness later. It's your decision.

An hour a day of straight cardio, or a full 60 minutes of straight weight machines, is hardly excessive, when you consider how inert your body is for much of the rest of your waking hours. Think about this, especially if you have a desk job, and especially if you watch a lot of TV. How much time do you spend sitting virtually still, reading, talking on the phone or surfing the Internet? All that sitting adds up. For optimum paybacks, you must balance your workouts with aerobic and anaerobic type exercise, as they each have something different to offer in terms of upgrading health and fitness. And don't just "go through the motions" while exercising; push yourself for continued improvement. For most of us, it's healthy to increase our heart rate, respiratory rate and sweat a little.

Aerobic/Cardio Exercise

This involves sustained activities that require stamina, such as jogging, swimming, cycling, "aerobics classes" or cardio videos, brisk walking, cross-country skiing, and use of cardio equipment.

Choosing the Right Cardio Activity

Treadmills

In terms of aerobic activities, treadmill walking ranks very high, providing low impact workouts with relatively little risk of injury. Newer treadmills feature surfaces that absorb impact and reduce pressure on critical regions such as the Achilles' tendon, ankles, knees, hips and the low back. Treadmills also provide versatility. Speed and incline can be tailored to a user's specifications. Most treadmills are also equipped with automatic heart rate monitors, allowing users to keep tabs on their target heart rate throughout the session.

The harm of holding onto the treadmill. Most new exercisers instinctively hold onto the machine's front rails. *This is fine for a temporary heart rate check.* But after you get a reading, let go. If the machine keeps telling you, "Hold on for heart rate," then select a program that doesn't nag about this. Walking is great exercise when performed the way the human body was designed to walk: with arms swinging at sides, and posture upright. If you hold onto the treadmill, you will disrupt spinal alignment, encourage forward posture and tight shoulders, and burn far fewer calories than the display panel shows.

Holding onto or "resting" your hands on the side rails is also bad news. Any kind of holding on has the potential to raise blood pressure at faster speeds. Also, at faster speeds, holding on can result in stress injuries to the hips. Clinging to the machine "unteaches" your body proper walking mechanics, and it worsens balance. This will not pay off in the real world, where there's nothing to hold onto and where you must balance as you walk on uneven surfaces!

If you're afraid of falling off, then start out slowly enough to eliminate this fear. Most treadmills go as slow as 1 mph. Then, gradually increase speed as you mentally adjust to the idea of walking on a moving tread. Hanging onto the machine while using the incline totally cancels out the incline's effect. If it's too difficult to let go, then this means either the tread is moving too fast for the angle, or the angle is too high for the speed! Slow down, and/or lower the incline. Find the settings that allow you to walk naturally, hands off, while still feeling challenged. Remember, holding on will never simulate actual walking, and can ruin posture.

Elliptical Trainers

Elliptical trainers combine the natural stride of walking and the simplicity of a stair climber. Motion studies have demonstrated that the human foot actually moves through an elliptical pattern as we walk, jog or run. Elliptical trainers are truly unique in that they have the ability to offer a weight-bearing workout that minimizes stress on the joints. There is virtually no impact, as the user's feet never leave the pedals. This makes elliptical trainers ideal for anyone with back, knee, hip or ankle problems.

Because elliptical trainers offer a weight-bearing workout, they help increase bone density. Never slump forward on the elliptical. This is a common problem: People grasp the machine's bars for dear life and slouch forward, butt sticking out. This cheats their abdominal area and lower back from participating in the workout, encourages bad posture and burns fewer calories than what the display shows. Keep your body erect and vertical at all times. Holding onto the machine should be limited to a few fingertips lightly making contact with the bars, rather than the entire hand wrapped around in a grip-hold. Since the elliptical motion is not as close to nature as treadmill walking, you will not sabotage efforts by keeping a *few fingertips lightly resting* on the bars, as long as your posture remains proper.

Don't Prefer Treadmill or Elliptical?

Join a health club and try out its many aerobics classes: Spinning, step, various dance forms, cardio-combo formats using light weights, "boot camp" classes, cardio kickboxing (using bags as targets), "light impact" cardio, and so on. Or join a martial arts school. Martial arts are cardio-based. Some schools offer classes just for seniors. Because martial arts schools always offer classes for beginners, you cannot use your age, excess body weight, or lack of coordination as an excuse for bypassing this artistic form of physical discipline. If you still haven't found something you can look forward to doing, venture a little bit outside the boundaries. Try hiking, inline skating, tennis, basketball, racquetball or even belly dancing.

Guidelines for Cardio Exercise

1. Begin with a slow 5-minute warm-up and end with a 5-minute cool-down period.
2. Be consistent!
3. In order to gain health benefits from aerobics, you should exercise briskly for a minimum of 30 minutes per day, five to six days per week. Housework never substitutes for these exercise periods! As your fitness level improves, increase the length of aerobic sessions to 45-60 minutes per day for optimal benefit.
4. If you are out-of-shape or elderly, begin with 5-10 minutes of low intensity activity every other day, and gradually build toward a goal of 30 minutes. Again, don't say to yourself, "I don't need to do my 10-minute walk today because I spent 45 minutes putting up wall-paper." Your time slot for cardio exercise is still open! Do not develop the bad habit of filling your exercise time slot with household chores.
5. If your schedule is tight, aerobic activity can be broken into two, 15-minute segments. But make them count, since 15 minutes isn't a lot of time. Again, do not stick those 15 minutes of washing the car and raking the leaves into your 15-minute exercise slot. Structured, deliberate exercise is an opportunity for your body to regain (or improve) good posture and proper spinal alignment during physical exertion. Housework or yard chores create imbalances in spinal alignment and can literally throw your back out of whack and strain shoulder tendons. Structured exercise will help readjust your body.

Going Through Mere Motions Won't Cut It

One of the biggest problems I've noticed at fitness centers and gyms is that many people "go through the motions" during aerobic activity. It's not uncommon to see people on treadmills or bikes reading a book or watching TV and not even breaking a sweat. They've hardly increased their heart rate one beat during the entire session and are simply wasting their time. Whether you seek to improve heart health, or lose excess body fat, you must exercise hard enough to increase your heart rate. Don't be afraid to break a sweat while exercising.

Heart Rate

In order to achieve the most from your aerobics sessions, you should exercise at an intensity level between 50-80 percent of your maximum heart rate (MHR).

Determine your MHR.

1. Subtract your age from 220. This is your estimated maximum heart rate—an estimation of how fast your heart can beat in one minute.
2. Next, multiply this number by .50 and by .80 to find your target heart range (THR).

For example: Elizabeth is a 20-year-old female planning to start an aerobic exercise program. Her calculations would be:

1. 220—20 (her age in years) = 200 beats per minute: the maximum number of times her heart can beat safely in one minute.
2. To determine her THR, multiply 200 by .50 (100 beats) and by .80 (160 beats).

Elizabeth's THR would be between 100 and 160 beats per minute. She should exercise at a pace vigorous enough to keep her heart rate (pulse) between 100 and 160 beats per minute.

Now that you understand how to obtain your MHR and THR, the next step is learning how to measure it during exercise. To do so, stop exercising and find your pulse using only your first two fingers (either at the neck or wrist), then count each pulse or beat for 15 seconds. Next, multiply this number by 4 to get your heart rate per minute (15 seconds x 4 equals one minute). If this number is below the lower limit of your THR, you need to exercise a little harder or faster. If it's above the upper limit of your THR, you'll need to slow down a bit. For best results, monitor your pulse periodically while exercising to stay within your target heart range. With a little practice, you'll know exactly how hard to exercise without having to stop and measure your pulse.

If you hate the thought of stopping exercise and performing calculations, you can use the American Heart Association's "conversational-pace" rule. Ideally you should attempt to exercise at a pace that makes it difficult to talk to the person next to you. If you can speak comfortably, then you're not exercising hard enough and need to increase your pace. If you can't get more than a few words out without gasping for air, you probably need to slow your pace a bit.

I recommend beginning at the lower portion of your target heart range and working your way up as your aerobic fitness level improves. Remember, it is the time you spend performing aerobic exercise that matters most, not the speed or intensity of the exercise. If you cannot last for 45-60 minutes during your aerobic session, you are probably exercising too hard and need to reduce the speed a little until your fitness level improves. If you currently suffer from severe heart disease or some other marked medical condition, you may require a medically supervised exercise program. Speak to your doctor if you fall into this category before beginning an exercise regimen.

Anaerobic ("Resistance") Exercise

This refers to activity that requires a high expenditure of energy for short periods of time. Examples include weight training, sprinting, basketball and football. For purposes of this discussion, when we speak of anaerobic exercise, we are referring to weight training—which is also commonly referred to as strength training or lifting weights.

While aerobic workouts build cardiovascular integrity, it is weight training that toughens bones and joints. Why just settle for a healthy heart while your shoulder joints go to pot? Weight routines are just as important for women as they are for men. While lifting weights does little for cardiovascular health, it is unbeatable when it comes to raising your resting metabolic rate. And this, in turn, results in fat loss.

Weight training is the only type of exercise that can actually slow down, or even reverse, the decline in muscle mass, bone density and strength that occur with aging. In fact, by the time people reach age 70, they have lost about 40 percent of their muscle mass, assuming they have led a sedentary lifestyle. These losses significantly increase a person's risk for falls, serious fractures, disability and even premature death. Other benefits of weight workouts include a leaner body and increased lean muscle mass, greater range of motion in joints, and higher energy levels. And as just mentioned, a most-desirable side effect of weight training is the faster basal metabolic rate, which means many more calories burned at rest.

You needn't spend hours a day in a gym hoisting around loads of weight. In fact, if you're just beginning, a weight-training program need only take about 10-15 minutes per day, three days per week, to be effective. But as you become more conditioned, you should strive for 45-60-minute sessions for optimal results. That may sound like a lot of time stressing the muscles, but don't forget what your muscles do the rest of the time you are awake: not much! Sitting at a desk all day, watering the houseplants, setting the table, loading the dishwasher, typing at your computer, flipping through a magazine and assisting your child with his art project do not require any kind of anaerobic work.

These simple guidelines will help get you started:

1. Work out with weights a minimum of three times weekly.
2. Allow at least 48 hours of rest between your workouts for full recovery (e.g., M-W-F or T-Th-S).
3. Train all major muscle groups during each workout. These are: chest, shoulders, back, biceps, triceps, quadriceps, hamstrings and abdominals.
4. Perform a minimum of one set of 8-12 repetitions for each muscle group or exercise.
5. Challenge yourself by using a weight that results in "near-fatigue" on the last one or two repetitions.
6. Rest 45-90 seconds between each set.
7. When you are able to perform 12 repetitions with ease, add more weight.
8. As your conditioning improves, increase the number of sets for each exercise up to a maximum of three sets.
9. If you require additional help or want to invest more time into working out, consider hiring a certified personal trainer who can tailor a strength-training program that suits your specific needs.

Below is a simple weight-training routine designed for beginners. This program should take only about 15 minutes to complete. The exercises here target all major muscle groups. This workout should be performed every other day, three times weekly.

EXERCISE	SETS	REPETITIONS	WEIGHT
Chest Press	1	8-12	Near Fatigue
Shoulder Press	1	8-12	Near Fatigue
Lat Pull-Downs	1	8-12	Near Fatigue
Biceps Curls	1	8-12	Near Fatigue
Triceps Pushdown	1	8-12	Near Fatigue
Leg Press or Squat	1	8-12	Near Fatigue
Leg Extension	1	8-12	Near Fatigue
Leg Curl	1	8-12	Near Fatigue
Abdominal Crunches	1	As many as possible	

Personal Training: What Are You Waiting For?

Many people cite price as the reason they won't hire a personal trainer. But how much do you spend on junk food every month? Cigarettes? Liquor? Clothes you don't need? CDs you'll tire of within 30 days? It all adds up. You have the money. It's just a matter of where you choose to put it. Though personal training isn't cheap, it's also not something to be equated with springing for a Cadillac, either.

Personal training is often offered in the form of package deals. An individual who thinks personal training is "too expensive" will think nothing of spending the same amount of money on a one-week cruise in which he or she will gain weight, and then after the venture is over and the person has nothing to show for it except more pudge in the middle and maybe a sunburn. Personal training is a smart investment, in which the effects can last a lifetime, with the right trainer.

Exercise Guidelines

The American College of Sports Medicine (ACSM) recommends that all individuals over the age of 35 have a stress test prior to beginning an exercise program. This decision is best left up to your doctor who can more accurately assess your risk factors and determine your need for such a test. In principle, there is clearly more risk associated with a sedentary lifestyle than with activity. The need for a thorough medical exam should be more so recommended for people who choose to live an inactive lifestyle. In any event, it's always a good idea to consult with your doctor before starting an exercise program for the first time, or when changing to a different regimen. This is especially true if you currently suffer from cardiovascular illness or a metabolic disease such as Type 2 diabetes.

If you are exercising and experience the following symptoms, consult your doctor immediately.

- Pain or pressure in the left or mid-chest area, left neck, left shoulder or left arm
- Frequent bouts of dizziness or loss of consciousness
- Shortness of breath after mild exertion
- Reoccurring chest pains within the last several months

Special note: It is common knowledge that before beginning an exercise program, the previously inactive adult should get clearance from a physician. It is highly unlikely that a medical doctor will tell a patient, "Do not exercise. It's bad for you. If you exercise, you'll get sick and shorten your life span." Obviously, the "clearance" pertains to *type* of exercise. For example, upon a medical evaluation, a doctor may determine that his patient has high blood pressure or brittle bone disease (osteoporosis). This patient desperately needs to exercise, to help bring down blood pressure, or to increase bone density. However, there are certain kinds of exercises—and exercise techniques—that this patient should avoid.

A doctor will not necessarily know what these exercises and techniques are, because physicians are trained in diagnosing and medically treating disease, not in designing exercise programs. Thus, a person with medical conditions should feel comfortable consulting with an experienced, certified personal trainer, particularly one who is certified in training people with the medical issues in question. Many trainers specialize in cardiac clients, for example. Some focus on the senior population, or on "special" populations—those needing a higher level of individualized design for their exercise program.

Genes Don't Doom You; Lifestyle Choices Do.

What's a greater predictor of life span? Genetic makeup, or how you live your life? A study appearing in the *Journal of the American Medical Association* (1998) found that when the genetic sample is controlled using twins, the effects of exercise are still apparent. Researchers studied a group of over 7,900 twins and found that those who exercised only six times per month for at least 30 minutes had a better chance of living a long life.

Exercise and Life Expectancy

Dr. Ralph Paffenbarger, an epidemiologist who has been researching the medical benefits of exercise for years, believes it can reduce our risk of death. In a study known as the Harvard Alumni Study, Dr. Paffenbarger and his associates carefully examined the activity levels of over 17,000 volunteers dating back to 1962. The results showed a strong inverse relationship between total physical activity and death from all causes. In other words, the more the volunteers exercised, the lower their risk of death became. The researchers concluded that the men who exercised regularly had a 23 percent lower risk of death than their sedentary counterparts.

In a Nutshell

Research has consistently demonstrated that people who keep their body fit are not only healthier, but also tend to live longer than those who do not. Studies have shown that death rates can be 25-33 percent lower among people who use 2,000 or more calories during exercise per week. Burning up 3,500 calories a week has been shown to lower death rates by up to 50 percent. Regular exercise increases life expectancy by reducing the risk of common diseases that contribute to premature death in the U.S.

These include heart disease, cancer, stroke, diabetes, hypertension, obesity and even Alzheimer's disease. Regular exercise will also help you look and feel your best throughout life. No medication on the market today can provide the health benefits associated with regular exercise. Exercise need not be strenuous to improve health and increase life expectancy. Research has found that how long you exercise may be more important than how hard or intense you exercise when it comes to the health of your heart. Your minimum goal for exercise should be 30 minutes of brisk aerobic type exercise five to six days per week, and three days a week of weight training. It's that simple.

Chapter 5 Goals:

- ✓ Commit to an exercise program that includes at least 30 minutes of *brisk* aerobic type exercise 5-6 days per week.
- ✓ Commit to three days a week of weight training.
- ✓ If need be, hire a personal trainer to help you design an exercise program that suits your individual needs and to help with motivation.

Chapter 6

Ideal Body Weight—Drop Those Excess Pounds Forever

Life Extension Value: 2-13 Years

Obesity is chomping down on tobacco as the top underlying cause of preventable death in America. This isn't hard to believe. Just look around at all the super-plus-sized people at any crowded event. At a zoo or amusement park, you won't have any problem spotting dozens of young kids who waddle rather than walk. And oftentimes, their parents are the size of houses.

Obesity can result in a heart attack that cuts a person's life way short at only age 50. Or, it can lead to cancer, which can lead to the same tragic result. But collectively, as a general population, just how many years of life do overweight people lose?

Researchers estimate that a 20-year-old white male with a body mass index (BMI) of 45 or more is predicted to die 13 years sooner than a 20-year-old who is not obese. A 20-year-old white woman with a BMI of 45 was estimated to lose about eight years of life. Even more moderate levels of obesity (BMI greater than 30) were shown to reduce life expectancy between 2-5 years for both men and women.

You may think a 2-5 year reduction isn't significant, but remember that obesity (even moderate levels) is most infamous for ruining the quality of a person's life. By genetic luck of the draw, a clinically obese person may live to be 85, but you can bet that many of those years—perhaps three or even four decades—were spent in a lot of pain, plus labored breathing from only mild activities, not to mention the inability to participate in many ventures.

Next time you see an obese person, who appears to be of great-grandparent age, realize that chances are pretty high that he or she must take a battery of drugs every day to manage a cluster of medical conditions brought on by obesity: Type 2 diabetes, osteoarthritis, high blood pressure, high cholesterol, heart disease, even gout. And it's highly probable that this individual has been living with multiple medical conditions (and thus pain) for many, many years. I've never known an obese, inactive 60-year-old who **didn't** have trouble getting into and out of cars.

The latest data from the National Center for Health Statistics show that an estimated 65 percent of adults are either overweight or obese, and an estimated 16 percent of children and adolescents are overweight. If you are already at your ideal body weight—congratulations—you have just earned yourself an extra 2-3 years of life!

Recent weight studies have shown the following associations between weight and life expectancy:

- People who are overweight (but not obese) are likely to suffer a reduced life span of between 2-5 years, compared to those of normal weight. Ever see a fat 100-year-old? 90-year-old? 80-year-old? If you've seen obese 80-year-olds, chances are, they were confined to wheelchairs or had considerable difficulty walking.
- Obese women have a reduced life span by 7.1 years.
- Obese men have a reduced life span by 5.8 years.
- Morbidly obese men—(at least 100 pounds overweight) have a reduced life span by up to 13 years.

Researchers have discovered that being overweight or obese increases the risk of many diseases and health conditions, including the following:

- Heart disease
- High blood pressure
- Stroke
- Certain cancers
- Type 2 diabetes
- Abnormal blood fats (cholesterol, triglycerides)
- Gallbladder disease
- Osteoarthritis
- Sleep apnea
- Chronic fatigue
- Depression
- Low self-esteem

Americans are digging their graves with eating utensils, gorging more than ever on junky foods, and spending more time sitting around. Remember when 8 ounces of soda used to quench your thirst? Now, ingenious marketing campaigns have convinced the public that 40 ounces are needed for the job. Thirty years ago, who would have thought you could get a chili cheese dog and nachos at a gas station? People fill up their cars, then go inside the shop to pay for the gas, and staring right at them at the pay counter are the brownies and cookies.

"Obesity" means being at least 20 percent over one's ideal body weight range. Body composition must also be taken into account. A person can have excess body fat yet not appear to be "overweight" at all as long as he's wearing a business suit. But if he were in swim trunks, you'd clearly see the extra fat in his stomach; and in women with high body fat levels—but not a big body—extra fat is often visible on the thighs. A size 8 doesn't always mean ideal body fat percentage. In general, a person with a weight problem can see it in the mirror.

The vast majority of overweight cases are caused by eating more food than your body burns off as fuel. The formula is relative. A person with a very slow metabolism who never exercises, doesn't have to eat that much to be overweight. And there are people who sweat hard two hours a day and are still 40 pounds overweight—-because they eat 8,000 calories a day.

Common causes of a slow metabolism are: lack of exercise, low muscle mass, poor eating habits and infrequent eating/skipping meals. Metabolism slows down as we age, but not directly from the aging process. It's from loss of muscle over time. A sedentary lifestyle results in muscle loss beginning at about age 30.

Should You Lose Weight?

Most people can tell if they need to lose weight just by standing in front of a mirror or by their clothing becoming tighter. But how can you determine if that spare tire is putting you at risk for illness and disease or is just an aesthetic concern?

One of the more common ways to determine if you are at an ideal body weight is through a body mass index (BMI) measurement, which is based on height and weight. To simplify, here is a link to an automated BMI calculator that I have posted on my website, along with several other automated tools designed to save you some time. You can access this link at: www.LongevityMadeEasy.com

A desirable BMI is between 18.5 and 24.99. An individual with a BMI of 25 to 29.99, or, who is between 25-30 lbs over recommended weight, is considered overweight (unless you are an athlete and have an increased lean body mass). An individual with a BMI of 30 or greater, or, who is at least 30 lbs over recommended body weight, is considered obese.

Also, just because you have a desirable BMI doesn't actually mean you are healthy. A thin person can still have life-threatening plaque caked on the inside of his or her arteries. If you—with your slim body—have poor dietary habits and lead an unhealthy lifestyle, you are still deep in the middle of the woods.

In addition to calculating your BMI, you can also use your waist-to-hip ratio (see below) to help assess your risk for future illness and disease. Several recent studies have demonstrated that the waist-to-hip ratio is a more accurate measure of obesity and a better predictor of heart attack risk than the body mass index.

A waist circumference of more than 32 inches in women and more than 34 inches in men is linked to an increased risk for heart attack. Men with a waist measurement of 40 or more inches are also 12 times as likely to develop diabetes as men with a waist measuring 29 to 34 inches. Remember, waist circumference is not the same as your waist-to-hip ratio. It's simply your waist size.

To determine your waist-to-hip ratio, measure your waist at its narrowest point (typically belly button), and measure your hips at their widest point with a tape measure. Below is a link to an automated waist-to-hip circumference calculator that I have posted on my website.

You can access that link at: www.LongevityMadeEasy.com

After determining your waist-to-hip circumference, you can check your result with the table below.

Male	Female	Risk
0.95 or below	0.80 or below	Low risk
0.96 to 1.0	0.81 to 0.85	Moderate risk
1.0 or greater	0.85 or greater	High risk

Barrel Shaped or Pear Shaped?

Where fat is stored on your body has major health implications and may lead to disaster. Individuals with more fat around their abdomen (spare tire) have an increased risk of high blood pressure, Type 2 diabetes, coronary artery disease and premature death—compared to equally hefty individuals but with more of their fat on the extremities.

Many Pregnancies Never an Excuse for Being Overweight

Nowhere in the annals of medical science does it state that experiencing multiple pregnancies causes permanent excess body fat. Fat cells do not permanently increase in size or quantity from pregnancies. The only agent that impacts the size of fat cells is calories in, versus calories out. Period.

Nevertheless, women often do gain quite a bit of weight during pregnancy. A weight gain of 25-35 pounds is normal. During pregnancy, a woman's metabolism actually increases. But at the same time, her appetite often increases, and her physical activity slows down. The net result is more body fat by the time the baby is born. But nothing intrinsic to the pregnancy causes the weight gain. The fat increase is the result of higher food consumption, and reduced physical activity. And that higher food consumption and diminished physical activity often persist long after the pregnancy is over.

Some women will blame a weight gain of 80 or even 100 pounds on having had several children, especially if a birth involved multiples. (In the case of multiples, a woman is often prescribed ongoing bed rest in the last trimester, and this inertia can cause substantial weight gain.) And it's a very observable phenomenon that many women indeed gain weight over the years—as more babies are born. The correlation between the arrival of more children, and the addition of more body fat, cannot be disputed.

But does this mean that having babies makes a woman "fat"? And what if the fat is still there, five years after the last birth? Is pregnancy supposed to "ruin" a woman's figure? Or is this just an old wives' tale? Let's examine some lifestyle changes that a growing family causes:

- Far less time to exercise. Gym sessions are skipped. Tennis matches are forfeited. Hikes are given up.
- The increased food consumption during pregnancy becomes a difficult habit to break, once the baby is born.
- Kids in the house mean more snacks in the house, more baking, and more food in general.
- A busy mother may end up eating food off her kids' plates, rather than hassling with preserving it. Those two remaining chicken nuggets and three tablespoons of potato salad can be very tempting, and end up in the mouth rather than in the Tupperware.
- The weight gain dampers a woman's spirits, and may fuel a desire to eat even more for solace. She may think there's no point in getting back into a strict exercise routine. The cycle is vicious. Lack of exercise means loss of muscle, which means slower metabolism, which means even more fat gain.
- Heart disease, Type 2 diabetes, stroke, cancer and joint problems don't give a hoot how many pregnancies you've had!

Why Fad Diets Fail and Can Predispose You to Disease

Fad diets come and go, but all seem to have a common theme. They appeal to the masses by making promises that sound too good to be true. Nearly all of these diets offer a quick—and unrealistic-solution to weight loss. Fad diets, and diets in general, have several problems. For one, the primary goal of most diets is rapid weight loss. They commonly restrict the individual to specific types of food, and promise miracle weight-loss results almost overnight (which doesn't make sense, when you consider that a person doesn't gain 50 or 100 pounds overnight). As a result, these diets tend to be nutritionally unbalanced and so boring that it's almost impossible to stay on them for long periods.

Low-Carb/High-Protein Diets

Low-carbohydrate diets tend to be high in protein and fat and deficient in key nutrients. The hazards associated with high protein, low carb plans are numerous, including:

- Bone loss
- Ketosis (an accumulation of toxic ketone bodies in the blood resulting from fat breakdown, which can cause nausea, vomiting, apathy, fatigue and low blood pressure)
- Gout
- Elevated cholesterol

Consuming excessive amounts of protein also forces your kidneys to get rid of large amounts of nitrogen wastes, resulting in frequent trips to the toilet, and the loss of large amounts of water. As a result, the weight lost from these diets is primarily water and not body fat. High carb, low protein diets can also lead to problems because your body is forced to "eat" its own muscle tissue for new protein. This lean body mass that you lose, actually burns fat and supplies strength.

Starvation Diets

These "trick" your body into thinking it's in the midst of a famine. To cope with this, your body holds onto stored fat, i.e., your metabolism becomes stunted. Because fad and starvation diets are nutritionally void, they can also put you at risk for illness and disease. Finally, they leave you hungry and feeling cheated out of a basic pleasure in life, making you more apt to binge sooner or later and tumble off the wagon.

Nutritional Supplements Aimed at Weight Loss

Ads for these products jam up radio air time, usually with a near-histrionic voice-over, or someone claiming to be a doctor pitching the virtues of "just one tablet a day." Magazines also carry these crazy ads, typically claiming that the pill melts fat while you sleep. Often, celebrities are used for these ads, as though the advertiser just knows that the gullible public will automatically think that the curvy blonde TV star in the ad really, truly uses the product. And unfortunately, many consumers fall for this ploy.

Because the FDA does not monitor supplements and herbs, there is no way of knowing a product's quality, safety and effectiveness. Some ads attempt to portray their herbal products as drugs with clever names and labels; magazine print ads show pictures of men in white jackets with stethoscopes. People desperate to lose unwanted pounds are further lured to these products by their risk-free offers and money-back guarantees. And is there a such thing as a weight loss pill that doesn't boast, "gives you energy!"?

Aside from all the gimmicks, most, if not all of the fat burners on the market today contain one or more of the following ingredients. Many of them also attempt to separate themselves from the competition by additional ingredients or by coming up with unique trademarked names for common ingredients.

Green Tea Extract
Verdict: Thumbs up

Studies published in the December 1999 issue of the *American Journal of Clinical Nutrition and Urology* show that substances abundant in green tea extracts may promote weight loss. Study participants were put on a diet consisting of about 13 percent protein, 40 percent fat and 47 percent carbohydrates. For six weeks, the men took either green tea extract plus caffeine; caffeine alone; or a placebo (sugar pill) with each meal. Results showed that the men taking the green tea extract experienced a significant increase in their 24-hour energy expenditure (the number of total calories burned in a 24-hour period) over those taking only caffeine or the placebo, and that they also burned more fat calories than those taking the placebo. There was no difference between caffeine users and placebo users in terms of fat calorie burning or overall calorie burning.

A second study recently published in the *American Journal of Clinical Nutrition* (2005) showed that people who drank tea fortified with green tea extract every day for three months lost more body fat than those who drank regular oolong tea. In this study, 35 Japanese men with similar weights and waist sizes were divided into two groups. For three months, the first group drank oolong tea fortified with green tea extract containing 690 milligrams of catechins, and the other group drank oolong tea with 22 milligrams of catechins (no extract added). During this time, the men ate identical breakfasts and dinners and were instructed to control their calorie and fat intake at all times so that overall total diets were similar.

After three months, the men who drank the green tea extract lost more weight (5.3 pounds) and experienced a significantly greater decrease in body mass index (BMI), waist size and total body fat. The catechin content varies by amount of green tea used and steeping time. But general recommendations, based on previous studies on the benefits of green tea, are at least four cups a day. Green tea extract supplements are also available. Green tea does not cause side effects. But caffeine-sensitive people may experience effects that are caffeine-related.

So here's what you need to know to protect yourself from being scammed. The dose of catechins, or EGCG, used in the previous study was about 700 milligrams. If you're taking a fat burner containing much less than this, you're wasting your money. If you're not following a healthy, low fat diet, don't expect results.

Rather than spending your money on a fat burner, I recommend going to your local nutrition outlet and purchasing green tea extract (liquid or capsule form) and taking it with a few cups of green tea each day. Just be sure to get the optimal daily dose of 700 mg catechins (EGCG).

Conjugated Linolenic Acid (CLA)
Verdict: Thumbs mostly up

CLA is a popular dietary supplement used, among other things, to promote weight loss and improve the ratio of fat to lean body mass. A study appearing in the *American Journal of Clinical Nutrition* (2005) reports that overweight patients given CLA (4,500 milligrams daily for 12 months) experienced weight loss and favorable changes in body composition. The most common side effects reported were gastrointestinal in nature. However, in a prior randomized trial in overweight humans, no benefits were seen after three months of consuming CLA. CLA can help with weight loss, but don't expect miracles. Without the right eating plan and exercise regimen, CLA will do little to improve your appearance or health.

Ephedra
Verdict: Thumbs up, with caution

Ephedra, also known as ma huang, is a strong herbal stimulant. Ephedra has been found to raise blood pressure and put stress on the circulatory system, and increasing stroke and heart attack risk. These dangers are thought to increase with dose, with strenuous activity and when ephedra is taken with caffeine.

The combination of ephedrine and caffeine is a potent and effective weight loss agent. Studies have shown that the combination of the two results in a monthly weight loss of about 2.2 pounds for up to 4-6 months' duration. I don't believe that ephedra is as dangerous as it's made out to be when used as directed. Problems begin to arise when individuals abuse the supplement, believing that "more is better," and that the more they take, the more weight they will lose. The American public is partly to blame for this ban <<is it currently banned? If so, why recommend it if people will have no access to it?>>because of irresponsible use of the herb and sole dependence on it as a primary agent for weight loss. After all, it's much easier to take some pills than it is to diet and exercise, right?

Caffeine
Verdict: Thumbs down

There have been a few studies published indicating that large amounts of caffeine—the equivalent of six cups of coffee per day—may slightly enhance weight loss in people who exercise regularly and who follow a low-fat diet. But there are no studies indicating that the weight lost from caffeine is significant or permanent. Caffeine does act as a diuretic and can lead to an increase in the amount of urine excreted. Furthermore, you will regain any water weight lost soon after you eat or drink.

Caffeine also acts as an appetite suppressant, but this effect lasts for only a short period and not long enough to contribute to significant weight loss. Keep in mind that caffeine is a stimulant and can increase heart rate and blood pressure, cause sleep disturbances and lead to nervousness and irritability in some people. Regular consumption of large amounts of caffeine can be detrimental to health.

Garcinia Cambogia—hydroxyl citric acid (HCA)
Verdict: Thumbs down

HCA, extracted from the Garcinia cambogia plant, has been studied extensively in animals and has been found to act as an appetite suppressant, and to modify their metabolism so that they have less of a tendency to convert carbohydrates to fat. The end result? The animals lost weight. So dietary supplement manufacturers took this information and ran with it.

Suddenly, HCA is the next miracle weight loss solution. The only problem is that HCA has not been proven to be an effective weight loss agent in studies involving human subjects. Several studies have shown that Garcinia cambogia failed to produce significant weight loss and fat loss beyond that observed with a placebo (sugar pill) in humans.

Despite these findings, HCA continues to appear in fat burners and is touted as an effective weight loss tool. The amount of HCA used per day in the study was 1,200 milligrams. I highly doubt that there are any fat burners on the market that contain more than a few hundred milligrams of HCA, further reducing the likelihood of any positive response.

Chromium Picolinate
Verdict: Thumbs down

A number of double-blind, placebo-controlled studies have reported on the effects of chromium supplementation and exercise on body composition in non-obese individuals. Two studies showed a greater effect on fat loss with supplementation, but have been criticized on methodological grounds. The remaining five showed no effect (*Nutr Rev* 1998; 56: 266-270.). Two further studies of obese individuals failed to show greater weight or fat loss with chromium supplementation (*Int J Obes* 1997; 21: 1143-1151) (*Med Sci Sports Exerc* 1997; 29: 992-998.). Even more troubling is the fact that chromium has been shown to accumulate in the tissues of humans and possibly causing irreversible damage to DNA (*FASEB J* 1995; 9: 1650-1657.). There have also been reports of renal damage following chronic ingestion of large doses of chromium picolinate. When it comes to chromium picolinate, the risks far outweigh the benefits.

L-Carnitine
Verdict: Thumbs down

L-carnitine is a common ingredient in many weight loss agents. Two studies have shown no changes in the rate of fat burning following L-carnitine supplementation (*Med Sci Sports Exerc* 1994; 26: 1122-1129) (*Am J Clin Nutr* 1990; 52: 889-894). At this time, there have been no controlled studies examining the effects of L-carnitine on weight loss that have been published.

Pyruvate
Verdict: Thumbs down

Pyruvate is a substance made in our bodies as a result of glucose metabolism. A study published in the *American Journal of Clinical Nutrition* (1992) showed that obese women who took pyruvate for three weeks lost 3.5 more pounds of body weight than a group given a placebo. This study did demonstrate that pyruvate may help certain people lose weight, but there's a catch. The participants in the study were taking 36,000 milligrams of pyruvate daily.

Because pyruvate is typically sold in 500 to 1,000 milligram capsules, you would have to take anywhere from 36-72 capsules a day to match the amount used in the study. The cost of pyruvate supplementation would be about \$15-\$20 per day, or more than \$400 over the course of three weeks to lose just over 3 lbs! Despite this, there are still products touting the benefits of pyruvate for weight loss. These products contain only a fraction of the amount used in the study, but the companies feel that it's enough to just include it in the product's list of ingredients.

Chitosan
Verdict: Thumbs down

Chitosan is made from chitin, which forms the shells of crabs, shrimp, lobsters, etc. It's similar to fiber, in that it passes through the intestinal system unabsorbed. Chitosan also takes a little recently consumed fat along with it for the ride, but it does nothing to remove the fat deposits already in your stomach or thighs. Although there is some evidence that chitosan was more effective than a placebo for short-term weight loss, many of the studies demonstrating weight loss with chitosan are of poor quality and contain inconsistent results.

The amount of weight loss from chitosan is minimal. Because chitosan binds and excretes fat that's consumed, it can also limit the absorption of fat-soluble vitamins (A, D, E, and K) and other valuable nutrients. Chitosan can also interfere with the absorption of some medications that are fat-soluble such as oral contraceptives and estrogen.

Guarana
Verdict: Thumbs down

Guarana is simply another form of caffeine. At this time, there are no studies that show guarana by itself can help with weight loss.

Bitter Orange
Verdict: Thumbs down

When the FDA banned ephedra in 2004, bitter orange extract quickly replaced ephedra as a prime ingredient in weight-loss products. The main active ingredient in bitter orange extract is synephrine. Synephrine has many of the adverse cardiovascular effects as ephedra. Because of its potential effects on the cardiovascular system, it may be especially dangerous when used by the elderly, the obese and those with high blood pressure or heart problems.

As you can see, there is little positive evidence that any of the ingredients reviewed here are effective in weight loss other than green tea extract (EGCG), and caffeine *when combined* with ephedra (side effects limit the use of this combination for most people). Many of the purported weight loss aids are very expensive and are a complete waste of your hard-earned dollars. Be an educated consumer and don't fall for these gimmicks. They simply do not work no matter what celebrity is touting their use.

Additional more detailed studies are needed before most of these products can be recommended for weight loss. I personally feel that of all the supplements mentioned, green tea extract is the only way to go. Not only is there a good amount of evidence supporting its use as a weight loss agent, more importantly, it has been found to have other positive health benefits. If you do decide to use green tea extract for weight reduction, I highly recommend purchasing the active ingredient (EGCG) and taking the effective dosage used in the studies (700 mg daily). Always keep in mind, of course, that lifestyle changes should be considered the basis of any weight loss initiative.

Secretly Fattening Foods

We are all aware that candy bars, cookies, cakes and sweetened soft drinks can contribute to weight gain, but many seemingly healthy foods can also lead to excess weight gain.

Limit or eliminate the following foods from your daily diet if you are having difficulty loosing weight:

1. Protein and energy bars
2. Nuts
3. Fruit smoothies
4. Dried fruit
5. Granola bars and cereal
6. Fruit juice
7. Specialty coffee drinks
8. Desserts labeled "non-fat" or "low-fat"

How to Lose Weight and Keep It Off

Here's the secret to losing weight and keeping it off. Burn more calories than you take in. It's really that simple. Now you're probably thinking, "It can't really be that simple." Well, I'm telling you that it really is as simple as that. If you spend more money than you deposit in your bank account, you will ultimately have less money in your account. Burn more gas than you put into your car, and you'll soon run out of gas. The same holds true for your body. It's simple mathematics.

So how do you burn more calories than you take in? By exercising more and making smarter decisions when it comes to meal planning. In other words, choosing foods that are nutritionally dense and low in calories. By switching from a diet of red meat, fried foods, sweetened beverages and baked goods to a plant-based diet, you are inadvertently reducing your daily caloric intake without actually reducing the quantity of food.

Now add in a brisk 30-45 minute walk most days of the week, and I guarantee you will lose weight and keep it off. In order to lose one pound of bodyweight, you have to use 3,500 more calories than you take in. If you take in 500 fewer calories per day by switching to a plant-based diet and burn an additional 500 calories per day through exercise, you will end up with a daily caloric deficit of 1,000 calories, or a weekly deficit of 7,000 calories—and lose 2 pounds per week.

The hardest part about weight loss is sticking to the program. That's not to say you can't enjoy a few scoops of ice cream, a slice of pizza or a chocolate bar on occasion. The key is not to make it a habit. I follow a healthy eating plan most days of the week and allow myself a "cheat" day to indulge in whatever I wish. When that day is over, it's right back to the healthy eating plan and regular exercise.

Guess what! I still look and feel great and have not gained any additional weight over the past 20 years except for lean muscle. I've never used a fad diet or relied on nutritional supplements aimed at weight loss—just a healthy eating plan and regular exercise. I've worked with hundreds of individuals over the years who have also had the same success using sound dietary habits and consistent exercise. You too can enjoy the same success if you simply dedicate yourself to a healthier lifestyle.

You will not find a specific diet plan spelled out in this section; they are useless. We all enjoy different foods and should not be forced to follow one specific plan of eating. In Chapter 5, you learned about my longevity "diet." I strongly believe that this is the healthiest eating plan you can follow, as it's nutritionally dense and naturally low in calories. Follow the guidelines outlined in the chapter and those in the chapter on exercise and you will lose all the weight you need to. Not only will you lose weight, your energy levels will improve dramatically as will your overall health and fitness level. Not only will you add years to your life, but life to your years!

Medical Causes of Weight Gain

Medical causes of extra fat are relatively very rare, in comparison to the general population of overweight people. For all practical purposes, the creation of the monster we call "fat" is rooted in our lifestyle. Evidence of this is in photos. View contemporary photos of throngs of people (not at a beach—beaches attract a lot of leaner people). Now, look at photos taken generations ago, of throngs of people. Check out photos taken at the turn of the century. The further you go back in time, the fewer fat people you see in the pictures. Nevertheless, some cases of obesity are clearly generated by medical circumstance.

- Thyroid disease
- Polycystic ovary syndrome (PCOS)
- Blood sugar abnormalities
- Cushing's syndrome
- Certain cancers
- Certain medication such as oral contraceptive pills, steroids, prednisone and anti-depressants

If you have attempted to lose weight with diet and exercise and have had little to no success, you may want to speak to your doctor about ordering a few simple tests that can help rule out a specific medical cause for weight gain. If everything turns up normal, take a sharper look at your eating and exercise habits. A sampling of just one tablespoon of gravy, to see if it's just right for the family dinner, is a hefty 100 calories. One Hershey Kiss is 30 calories. A little here, a little there...it all adds up. And strolling about the neighborhood won't shed the fat nearly as much as will a fast-paced, arm-swinging walk.

When It Comes to Bodyweight, Thinner is Always Better, Right?

Wrong. We are all aware than being overweight or obese is danger-ous to your health and well-being, but the same can hold true if you weigh too little. Many people are under the false assumption that thin-ner is always better. We are all surrounded by images of models and celebrities who are underweight. Unfortunately, many people (espe-cially women) compare themselves with others rather than by objec-tive standards when assessing their weight.

Many people who are underweight suffer from eating disorders. These eating disorders can put you at risk for a number of nutritional deficiencies. The health risks of eating disorders range from dry skin and brittle nails to anemia (fatigue), infertility, osteoporosis, cardiovas-cular damage, neurological complications and even death.

One of the more common eating disorders is anorexia nervosa. People with anorexia have an irrational fear of gaining weight despite weighing much less than others of the same height—sometimes liter-ally being skin and bones. So how do you know if you are under-weight? The easiest method for most people is a body mass index (BMI) calculation. Your BMI is based on your height and weight. A BMI of less than 18.5 can indicate that you are underweight and at risk for health problems. You can use my automated BMI calculator to determine yours (see BMI above).

A Serious Thought to Consider: Many people who wish to lose weight do not have the support of their family. If you are suffering with this problem, then you must stop perceiving it as a "problem" and forge ahead with making your weight goals a reality, never mind that some family members don't "support" you. When we are born, we don't come with a legal contract binding us to support family mem-bers when they wish to lose weight.

So if your family members, including spouse, don't "support" you, then stop depending on them to provide you with motivation. It's *your* body. You're the one who lives inside of it. Nobody else does. If an emotional support system is important to you, then don't seek it from discouraging people, even if they are family members. Instead, get it from a support group just for people working on losing weight.

There are no secrets here. It simply comes down to a will to succeed. If you are not totally committed to losing the weight, it's unlikely you will succeed. Follow my dietary and exercise recommendations and I'll guarantee you will not only lose the weight you want, but more importantly, you'll feel livelier and stronger than you've felt in years.

Chapter 6 Goals:

- ✓ Use the body mass index (BMI) and waist-to-hip ratio calculators to determine your ideal body weight. If you fall above or below this range, take the necessary steps described in this book to achieve and maintain a healthy weight.
- ✓ Do not rely on nutritional supplements for weight reduction.

Chapter 7

Sleep Your Way to Better Health

Life Extension Value: 9 Years

"Health is the first muse, and sleep is the condition to produce it."
—Ralph Waldo Emerson

Why do we need sleep in the first place? Sleep scientists aren't really sure. One theory suggests that early man acquired the need for sleep to quickly pass night time, which was scary during the cave-dwelling era, what with complete darkness and the sounds of wild animals nearby. This theory is weak because even primitive animals that are without fear have sleep cycles.

Another theory surmises that sleep developed to provide people with dreams. The dream stage of sleep is necessary for mental well-being. In studies in which people are deprived of the dream stage of sleep, they report excessive irritability and lack of concentration throughout the day. But this theory too is weak because even animals with very little free-will brain activity (i.e., animals whose actions are governed by instinct rather than choice and decision making) go to sleep every night. And yet another theory is based on common sense: The human body and mind simply need to fall asleep to rejuvenate for the next day.

But when was the last time that you awakened feeling rested, energized and alert? Most of us just don't get the sleep we need. We wake up drowsy, tired, achy and groggy. As we try to cram more and more activities and accomplishments into each day, we end up sacrificing the quality of our sleep, and ultimately our health. Sleep, like diet and exercise, is essential for our minds and bodies to function optimally.

Pretty much everyone has had the experience of awakening several times during the night, or too early, or lying in bed for hours unable to fall asleep. When these scenarios repeat themselves and disrupted sleep becomes a way of life, it can wreak havoc on mind and body. If you truly want to bring about optimal health, then you must begin to recognize the importance of sleep.

Effects of chronic sleep deprivation (6.5 hours or less of sleep per night) include:

- Slowed metabolism leading to weight gain
- Increased production of the stress hormone cortisol
- Decreased ability to secrete and respond to the hormone melatonin

---

What Research Tells Us About Sleep

A study published in the *British Medical Journal* found that a habitual routine of sleep deprivation causes metabolic and hormonal changes seen only in the elderly. Researchers now believe that many of these changes accelerate the aging process and are responsible for a variety of diseases and conditions.

Medical Conditions Linked to Sleep Deprivation

Heart Disease and Stroke

A 10-year study found that women who slept five hours or less per night had a 45 percent increased risk of developing heart disease, while those who slept nine or more hours a night had a 38 percent greater risk (sleeping too much can also be detrimental to your health). The same may also hold true for men.

Cancer

Sleep problems may increase the risk of certain cancers by altering the balance of two hormones in the body, cortisol and melatonin, and by disrupting the body's circadian rhythms. High levels of cortisol can depress the immune system. Melatonin, a hormone with antioxidant properties that is produced by the brain during sleep, is thought to help protect cells from damage that can lead to cancer.

In a study comparing blind women with sighted women, blind women had a 36 percent lower risk of breast cancer than the sighted women. Researchers at the Cancer Registry of Norway followed breast cancer incidence in over 15,000 visually impaired women, of whom 400 were completely blind. Totally blind women had a 36 percent lower risk of the disease compared to sighted women, according to a report in the *British Journal of Cancer* (2001; 84:397-399).

Amazingly, this lower incidence was not present among the women who were merely visually impaired but not totally blind. It is believed that exposure to artificial light at night (it's unnatural to be awake and up and about in the middle of the night) disrupts the natural melatonin-estrogen balance, resulting in less melatonin than there should be, and more estrogen. According to the analysis in this study, the result is a heightened risk of estrogen-sensitive tumors, like breast cancer.

So if you're a night worker who's been considering switching to days, perhaps you now have a very powerful incentive to finally do it. Sleeping in total darkness ensures optimal levels of melatonin and possibly reduces the risk for certain cancers. Individuals who often have disrupted sleep patterns from performing shift work also appear to have an increased susceptibility for cancer.

Data gathered from the Nurses' Health Study suggest that working a rotating night shift at least three nights per month for 15 or more years may increase the risk of colorectal cancer in women. This study supports earlier research that found women who work night shifts have a higher risk of breast cancer. On an individual level, women who worked a night shift rotation for at least 15 years had a 51 percent greater risk of rectum cancer, 41 percent greater risk of right colon cancer, and 22 percent greater risk of left colon cancer, compared to women who never worked rotating night shifts. (*J Natl Cancer Inst.* 2003 Jun 4; 95(11):825-8).

When the data linking breast cancer to shift work was revealed, people believed that higher estrogen levels resulting from melatonin suppression drove up the cancer risk. Melatonin has a tumor-inhibiting effect in laboratory tests. Colorectal cancer patients may have lower plasma levels of melatonin compared to healthy people. Thus, it may be melatonin, and not estrogen, that is influencing cancer risk, according to lead study author Eva S. Schernhammer, MD, of Harvard Medical School. "If melatonin's anti-cancer properties are the source of our observed effects, this research opens a whole new arena of potential associations between exposure to light and a variety of cancers."

Diabetes

In sleep-deprived individuals, blood sugar levels take 40 percent longer to drop following a high-carbohydrate meal. Other studies have found a 34 percent increase in diabetic symptoms in those getting less than 5 hours of sleep per night. Sleeping too much can also increase your risk for diabetic symptoms.

Obesity

An individual's risk for obesity increases with six or less hours of sleep per night. Sleep deprivation activates the appetite control center in the brain and influences the hormones leptin and ghrelin, both of which promote hunger. The body also sees sleep deprivation as a state of stress; cortisol is the stress hormone. Cortisol causes, in turn, the release of insulin, and insulin is a storage hormone that promotes fat storage.

According to a report published in the *Journal of the American Medical Association*, sleep problems can also complicate a variety of illnesses including Parkinson's disease, Alzheimer's disease, multiple sclerosis, gastrointestinal disorders, kidney disease and behavior problems in children.

Spending less time in deep sleep lowers production of growth hormone (GH). Signs and symptoms of low GH include reduced stamina, difficulty losing weight, reduced muscle mass, poor muscular strength and reduced libido. Positive effects of increased levels of GH include increased muscle mass, increased fat loss, improved skin texture, greater exercise tolerance, increased bone density, improved sleep quality and enhanced mental processes.

Growth Hormone: Get It From Sleep? Or Get It From a Pill?

Many people are under the false assumption that growth hormone can be administered as a pill, nasal spray or homoeopathic solution. The only way to receive growth hormone is through expensive injections. Companies now market so-called growth hormone stimulators that contain amino acids that supposedly boost the body's natural production of growth hormone. Absolutely no reliable evidence indicates that these supplements work. Save your hard-earned dollars when it comes to these products.

Circadian Rhythms and Your Body's Internal "Clock"

Circadian rhythms help regulate our sleep/wake cycles and energy levels, and also govern when hormones are released and other biological processes occur. Our bodies' "internal clock" controls these rhythms that last approximately 24 hours. This clock helps regulate our daily sleep patterns and is pre-programmed to make us feel sleepy at night and to be active during the daylight hours. It is also responsible for the production and secretion of growth hormone, cortisol and melatonin. The natural human biorhythm is to sleep between 10 pm and 6 am, meaning that ideally you should be in bed by 10 pm and up by 6 am. Research has shown that turning in before 11 pm induces better sleep.

The hormone melatonin is the primary controller of circadian (day/night) biorhythms. Melatonin is made in the pineal gland of the brain. Recent studies indicate that it may also be the central regulator of the hormonal component of the aging process. Normally, melatonin levels begin to rise in the mid-to-late evening, remain high for most of the night, and then slowly decline during the early morning hours.

Natural melatonin production is partially affected by light. Bright light suppresses the output of melatonin. When animals are exposed to light, their melatonin levels plummet immediately, almost as if a switch has been thrown. During the shorter days of the winter months, melatonin production can start earlier due to the increased darkness and in some people lead to symptoms of seasonal affective disorder (SAD). Melatonin levels also decline gradually with age. Some older adults produce very little amounts of melatonin or none at all.

So why exactly is melatonin so important to our well-being? Melatonin is a powerful antioxidant; more importantly, it is one of the few antioxidants that can actually penetrate into the cell's mitochondria. The mitochondria is the energy-producing part of a cell that contains its own DNA. The fact that nearly all of the antioxidants in nutritional supplements do not enter the mitochondria is believed to be the main reason that supplemental antioxidants do not noticeably extend life span and only minimally slow the aging process. Melatonin does appear to protect the mitochondria from oxidation damage.

As mentioned above, a number of animal studies have shown that melatonin reduces the incidence of some types of cancer, especially estrogen-mediated tumors such as breast cancer. In laboratory mice, oral melatonin supplementation increased life span to 931 days compared to a life span of 755 days for mice on an identical regimen without supplemental melatonin. Could these findings apply to humans as well? We're not sure, but studies are underway to help unravel the mystery of melatonin.

Remember, exposure to light during the sleep cycle, whether from a television, nightlight or bathroom light can reduce melatonin levels. Even the light coming in from an outdoor street-light can interfere. This is why it is absolutely essential that you do your best to sleep in total darkness.

Disruption of the body's circadian rhythms can lead to a variety of conditions including:

- Cardiovascular disease
- Cancer
- Diabetes
- Gastrointestinal problems
- High blood pressure
- Insomnia
- Depression
- Increased daytime sleepiness
- Decreased performance, both physical and mental
- Poor concentration
- Reduced productivity
- Impaired memory (forgetfulness) and reasoning
- Fatigue
- Irritability, frequent mood shifts and depression
- Increased stress

So How Much Sleep Do We Really Need?

According to the National Sleep Foundation, one third of adults don't keep regular sleep schedules, 21 percent have a caffeinated drink at night, and 90 percent report watching TV or listening to the radio in the hour before bedtime. Sleeplessness could be the result of medical problems; but chances are, it's self-imposed. Emerging research now tells us that for optimal health, most adults require about seven hours of quality sleep per night.

Common Causes of Sleep Disturbance

Stress is the top cause of short-term sleeping difficulties. Drinking alcohol or beverages containing caffeine in the evening, exercising close to bedtime, following an irregular morning and nighttime schedule, and working or doing other mentally intense activities right before or after getting into bed (such as working on a crossword puzzle) can disrupt sleep. Traveling also disturbs sleep, especially jet lag and traveling across several time zones; this can upset your biological or circadian rhythms.

Other environmental factors, such as a room that's too hot, too cold or too noisy, can cause sleep interference. Other influences to pay attention to are the comfort and size of your bed and the habits of your sleep partner. If you have to lie beside someone who snores, or who can't fall or stay asleep, has different sleep preferences or other sleep difficulties, it often becomes your problem, too. Finally, certain medications such as decongestants, corticosteroids, and some medicines for high blood pressure, asthma or depression can cause sleeping difficulties as a side effect.

Snoring: Sign of Potentially Fatal Condition

If you snore and experience other signs of disrupted sleep like excessive daytime sleepiness, you may be suffering from sleep apnea. Sleep apnea is a dangerous sleep disorder that typically worsens with age. Not only does sleep apnea result in sleep deprivation, but it can also threaten your life. This is because this disorder causes a person to stop breathing periodically during sleep. Some sufferers may stop breathing for as long as two minutes.

Sufferers have an obstructed airway due to relaxation and enlargement of the throat and tongue muscles, which cause them to awaken frequently in order to restart the breathing process. The frequency of waking episodes can vary, but they usually occur between 10 and 60 times per night, and up to 100-400 times in severe cases. In nearly all cases, individuals suffering from sleep apnea remember little to nothing of the waking episodes.

Signs and symptoms of sleep apnea include:

- Disrupted breathing, gasping, gagging or choking for air during sleep
- Loud snoring
- Feeling non-refreshed in the morning after a full night's sleep
- Daytime sleepiness/headaches/racing heart
- Lethargy
- Memory loss and difficulty concentrating
- Reduced attention span
- Personality changes

Ignoring the symptoms of sleep apnea can lead to serious health consequences including increased risk of sudden death, heart disease, stroke, high blood pressure and diabetes. Sleep apnea has also been linked to rapid weight gain and obesity, depression, impotence and reduced libido.

Treatment of Sleep Apnea

Common treatments for mild sleep apnea include weight loss; eliminating the use of alcohol, tobacco and sedatives; sleeping on your side; and normalizing your sleep patterns. Oral mouth devices that help keep the airway open may help reduce snoring in three different ways. Most treatment for moderate to severe sleep apnea involves C-PAP (continuous positive airway pressure). C-PAP is a machine that blows air into your nose via a nose mask, keeping the airway open and unobstructed.

The Plan for Improving Your Quality of Sleep

1. Maintain the same sleep schedule every day, including weekends. This helps set your body's internal clock. Avoid sleeping late on weekends; this only serves to disrupt sleep patterns.

2. Create an environment that is conducive to sleep. This may include adjusting room temperature, blocking out any light or noise, and selecting a comfortable mattress and pillow. If outdoor noise is a problem, invest in a soundproofing window.

3. Avoid consuming caffeine at least four to six hours prior to bedtime. The National Sleep Foundation reports that the effects of caffeine can lead to sleep problems in some people for as much as 10-12 hours after consumption. Also beware of over-the-counter drugs such as cold and cough preparations, which often contain caffeine.

4. Avoid consuming an excess of fluids before bed as they can awaken you through the night, causing you to run to the bathroom.

5. Quit smoking. Nicotine is linked to insomnia.

6. Avoid spicy and acidic foods before bed; they can lead to heartburn.

7. If you are having difficulty falling asleep, a glass of skim or low-fat milk before bed may be of benefit.

8. One more reason to commit yourself to exercise (morning or earlier in the day ideally): A fit body sleeps better.

9. Continual practice of the relaxation techniques described in Chapter 2 will improve sleep quality.

10. Channel your thoughts. Focus on something absorbing yet mechanical, such as counting backwards from 1,000 in increments of 18.

11. Avoid shift work, if possible.

12. If you are unable to fall asleep after 30 minutes, leave the room and engage in a quiet activity for a few minutes.

13. Avoid napping during the day if you have the time to sleep at night. If your job limits the amount of time for sleep, a nap may help restore energy and brainpower.

14. Prescription drugs such as beta-blockers, steroids, antidepressants, diuretics, bronchodilators and cholesterol-lowering medications can interfere with sleep. Speak to your doctor about switching medications.

If you continue to experience sleep difficulties after addressing these potential causes of sleep disturbance, you may require additional help.

Here are some of the more common treatments available for sleep disturbance.

Medications

The National Sleep Foundation provides the following guidelines for the use of medications to treat insomnia:

- The cause of insomnia has been identified and is best treated with medication.
- Sleep difficulties cause problems in accomplishing daily activities.
- Behavioral approaches have proven ineffective or the person is unwilling to try them.
- A person is suffering insomnia-related distress and beginning behavioral therapy.
- Insomnia is temporary or short-term.
- Insomnia is expected or occurs in association with a known medical or biological condition (e.g., premenstrual syndrome), or an event such as giving a speech or traveling across time zones.

Treatment with medications should:

- Begin with the lowest possible effective dose.
- Be short-term, if used nightly.
- Be intermittent if used long-term.
- Be used only in combination with good sleep practices and/or behavioral approaches.

It is very important that you work with your doctor to try to identify the cause and type of your insomnia before considering the use of medication. The best treatment for short-term insomnia that is linked to a specific stress or situation in your life is to address the situation and attempt to reduce the stress through behavioral modifications.

OTC sleep medications should be used for short-term insomnia only and in conjunction with changes to your sleeping habits.

Melatonin Supplementation

As dusk falls, the pineal gland in the brain secretes melatonin, tapering off towards dawn. Melatonin doesn't cause sleep, but it seems to initiate changes throughout the body that help prepare it for sleep.

Melatonin can also be of help to older adults, whose hormone production has slowed as a natural consequence of aging. However, melatonin isn't likely to help people who fall asleep easily but then wake up halfway through the night and can't get back to sleep again—the group that comprises the majority of insomniacs. Research from the U.S. Agency for Healthcare Research and Quality concluded that although melatonin helped insomniacs fall asleep faster when they got into bed, it didn't help them stay asleep or have restful sleep—making it an ineffective insomnia treatment overall.

If you opt for melatonin, begin with 1.5 mg daily, taken one hour or less before bedtime. If this dose is not effective, gradually increase dosage until an effective level is reached (up to 5 mg daily). There is research to suggest that synthetic melatonin may be safer than melatonin from animal sources.

5-HTP (5-hydroxytryptophan)

5-HTP is converted to serotonin in the brain. Serotonin is a neurotransmitter that influences sleep, body temperature, mood and behavior. Clinical trials show that 5-HTP is a safe, natural way to boost the brain's serotonin levels. 5-HTP increases REM sleep (dream stage) significantly while simultaneously increasing deep sleep stages 3 and 4 without increasing total sleep time. 5-HTP accomplishes this by shortening the amount of time you spend in sleep stages 1 and 2, which in certain ways are the least important stages of the cycle.

Dosage: 100 to 300 mg, 30-45 minutes before retiring. Start with the lower dose for at least three days, and increase if results are not achieved.

Melatonin vs. 5-HTP

5-HTP bypasses the brain's light-regulation system that controls the secretion of melatonin. Thus, when you take 5-HTP, it causes the release of melatonin irrespective of how much light is present.

People with low melatonin who take 5-HTP at nighttime can enjoy the same sleep enhancing benefits as they will from taking melatonin alone, but they will also be getting the broader spectrum of benefits that comes from increased serotonin levels. Melatonin alone does not enhance the functions of the serotonin system. People who use melatonin as a sleep sedative may find that switching from melatonin to 5-HTP will make it easier to fall asleep and to stay asleep.

Valerian

Valerian root is used in the traditional medicine of many cultures as a mild sedative and to aid the induction of sleep. Multiple compounds in valerian root have pharmacologic activity. Valerian has been demonstrated to decrease sleep onset time and promote deeper sleep. It improves the subjective experiences of sleep when taken nightly over a one-to two-week period and appears to be a safe sedative-hypnotic in patients with mild to moderate insomnia.

There are very few reported mild side effects of Valerian (such as dizziness and headache), and it is very well-tolerated for up to six weeks. To be effective, it has to be used in sufficiently high dosage.

For most people a single evening dose of valerian root extract (150-300 mg), 30 to 60 minutes before bedtime should suffice. It may take up to two weeks before the effects are felt. Valerian products should be standardized to contain 0.8 percent valerenic or valeric acid. For best results, purchase pure valerian root extract and avoid formulas containing multiple herbs.

Once sleep improves, valerian should be continued for two to four weeks. A total of four to six weeks is usually the length of treatment advised by herbalists. After six weeks, a two-week break is recommended to see if sleep has improved. Note: On very rare occasions, stopping causes withdrawal symptoms. Therefore, it's important to follow the directions of your healthcare practitioner when weaning off of valerian.

Cognitive Behavior Therapy

Cognitive behavioral therapy teaches people to recognize and change patterns of thought and behavior to solve their problems. Recently this type of therapy has proven very effective in getting people to fall asleep and conquer insomnia.

According to a study published in the *Archives of Internal Medicine*, cognitive behavior therapy is more effective at reducing insomnia and lasts longer than the widely used sleeping pill Ambien. When insomnia exists along with other psychological disorders like depression, experts agree that the initial treatment should address the underlying condition.

In a Nutshell

Sleep, like diet and exercise, is essential for good health. Emerging research now tells us that for optimal health, most adults require 7-8 hours of quality sleep per night. Chronic sleep deprivation or frequent sleep disturbance can adversely affect your health and has been linked to the development of heart disease, cancer, stroke, diabetes, obesity and premature aging. Other conditions linked to chronic sleep deprivation include hypertension, depression, increased daytime sleepiness, poor concentration, impaired memory and reasoning, and mood disorders. Sleeping more than necessary (eight-plus hours) can also be detrimental to your health.

Make yourself a commitment to get 7-8 hours of quality sleep each night. If you currently suffer from a sleep disorder, follow the recommendations in this chapter to improve the quality of your sleep. If these measures fail, speak to your doctor about prescribing a sleep aid. If you have reason to suspect that you suffer from sleep apnea, a potentially fatal condition, see your doctor immediately. Researchers have linked chronic sleep deprivation and sleep disturbance to a reduced life expectancy of 9 years! As you can see, not getting enough sleep can indeed kill you.

Chapter 7 Goals:

- ✓ Recognize the importance of sleep for overall health and well-being.
- ✓ Strive to get 7-8 hours of quality sleep per night.
- ✓ If you currently suffer from sleep disturbance, follow the recommendations outlined in this section to improve sleep quality or speak to your doctor about the use of prescription sleep aids.

Chapter 8

Supplements That Can Extend Your Life

Life Extension Value: 3 Years

Walk into any vitamin store or peruse the vitamin aisles in your drugstore and you will very likely become overwhelmed by literally thousands of nutritional products. Which ones are right for you? Which supplements bring on real benefits? This chapter will take the confusion out of nutritional supplementation. Good science has validated several specific supplements. These are the essential supplements needed to maintain or improve your health and give you the best shot at longevity.

Supplements, however, should play only a supporting role in your health; dietary sources should play the primary role. Do not dismiss the dietary guidelines from the previous phase and replace them with supplements. Nutritional supplements cannot erase damage caused by a poor diet and a sedentary lifestyle.

Of course, people don't always eat properly. A *USA Today* poll (2004) found that 85 percent of Americans don't get the recommended vegetable intake of five servings per day. As you already know, fruits and vegetables provide our primary source of nutrients and free radical fighting antioxidants. Supplementing your healthful diet with the nutrients recommended in this phase will keep you on track for a long and healthy life.

What Good Science Reveals About Supplements

A Daily Multivitamin/Mineral Supplement

In the June 19th, 2004, issue of the *Journal of the American Medical Association*, Harvard researchers recommend that all adults take a multivitamin supplement with minerals on a daily basis. The researchers made their recommendations on several key observations, including evidence linking suboptimal intakes of certain vitamins with an increased risk of chronic diseases.

A daily multivitamin will help offset the health risks associated with inadequate diet. One study estimated the potential preventative health benefits of multivitamin supplementation in the elderly at $1.6 billion over the following five years. Authors of the study calculated these savings on improved immune functioning and a reduction in the relative risk of coronary artery disease. Taking a daily multivitamin may also help protect against damage caused by free radicals. No scientific data has demonstrated harm in taking a daily multivitamin, so safety should not be a concern.

When choosing a multivitamin formula, be sure it contains a minimum of 100 percent of the daily values for each nutrient. Additionally, choose a multivitamin with minerals, since most Americans tend to be deficient as a result of depleted mineral stores in the soil and extensive refinement of food. To maximize absorption, take your daily multivitamin/mineral supplement with a meal, preferably breakfast.

10,000 Hits a Day (No, Not a Popular Website; Rather, Your Cells)

The term "antioxidant" refers to a group of naturally occurring substances that counteract the harmful effects of free radicals: highly reactive, toxic substances produced in the body during normal bodily functions such as respiration and metabolism. Exposure to environmental pollutants such as smog, sun, heavy metals, tobacco smoke, pesticides, over-the-counter medications and prescription drug interactions can also increase free radical production.

Additionally, factors such as regular exercise and a high fat diet have also been found to produce free radicals. In fact, as you are reading this book, millions of free radical attacks are occurring in your body. Biochemists have estimated that free radicals roaming the body hit every cell more than 10,000 times per day.

If left unchallenged, free radicals can cause irreversible damage to your body, and are implicated in over 60 different health conditions, including Alzheimer's. Increasing your daily intake of antioxidants can help limit the amount of damage caused by these renegade substances.

The addition of antioxidant supplements could especially benefit those who have inadequate diets. Data supporting the use of antioxidant supplements has been mixed, however; while some studies have demonstrated little to no benefit from supplementation, others have found significant benefits to their use. The greatest amount of evidence exists for the use of antioxidant supplements in the treatment of heart disease and certain cancers.

Primary Antioxidants:

- Vitamin C
- Vitamin E
- Selenium
- Beta-carotene (mixed carotenoids)
- Zinc

"Enriching" Antioxidants:

- Proanthocyanidins (including flavonoids, such as grape seed extract and pine bark)
- N-acetylcysteine
- Alpha-lipoic acid
- Coenzyme Q10
- Green tea extract

Antioxidants and Heart Disease

Antioxidants protect against heart disease by improving cholesterol profile. When LDL cholesterol comes in contact with free radicals in the body, it oxidizes and causes damage to the inside lining of the arteries. This damage accelerates the process of plaque formation within the arteries, causing them to narrow and, in turn, reduce blood flow to the heart. If blood flow is completely interrupted, a heart attack occurs.

Two studies published in the prestigious *New England Journal of Medicine* found that both men and women who took a daily vitamin E supplement for a minimum of two years, had a 37-41 percent reduced risk of heart disease. Results of the Cambridge Heart Antioxidant Study found a 75 percent reduction in the rate of nonfatal heart attacks in patients receiving vitamin E supplements after only one year of treatment. Vitamin E supplementation can help reduce C-reactive protein levels by 30 percent and in turn, may help reduce your risk for heart disease.

Are Vitamin E Supplements Safe?

A recent analysis linked vitamin E supplements to an increased risk of death. Many of the studies examined in this analysis included elderly people who had severe health problems. There is no way of knowing if these same findings would apply to healthy people. Several well-designed studies have found benefit from vitamin E supplements and as a result, I will continue to recommend them.

Add vitamin E to C for a mighty synergistic effect. These two vitamins go hand in hand, like two best buddies roaming inside your body, tidying up arteries, bringing down cholesterol, and just in general, promoting quality heart health. Vitamins E and C, when taken together, may lower heart attack risk.

According to a 1996 study published in the *American Journal of Clinical Nutrition*, daily intake of vitamin E supplements reduced the risk of heart attack by 47 percent, and when a daily dose of vitamin C supplements was added, the risk was reduced further to 53 percent. Vitamin C supplements have also been shown to improve arterial function in people with CAD, elevated cholesterol levels and chronic heart failure.

Selenium, an essential trace mineral, plays an important role in the etiology of cardiovascular disease and certain types of cancer.

Selenium, like vitamins E and C, helps limit oxidative damage to LDL ("bad") cholesterol in the blood. An increased risk of heart disease and certain cancers has been associated with reduced concentrations of selenium in the blood. It is difficult to obtain an adequate dose of selenium from dietary sources due to depleted concentration in the soil and processing of food, so I recommend a selenium supplement.

Antioxidants and Cancer

The prevalence of cancer has grown so rapidly in the American population, that for many people it is no longer a question of "if" they'll get it, but "when." Men have a 50 percent lifetime risk of developing cancer, and women face a 33 percent risk. The majority of all cancers found in humans are considered to be a result of lifestyle patterns such as exposure to tobacco smoke, and poor eating habits.

Free radicals play a role in the development of most cancers. Free radicals mangle up DNA and damage cells. In other words, the higher the antioxidant levels in your blood, the lower the incidence of cancer. Researchers believe that antioxidants inhibit the initiation of tumors, and can prevent cancer-causing compounds from reaching target sites in the body. Antioxidants can also beef up the body's own natural defense systems against cancer, and may help prevent or limit the spread of previously initiated cancers.

Researchers have conducted numerous studies on the potential of vitamin E to both prevent and treat certain types of cancers including those of the mouth, lung, colon, rectum, cervix, prostate and breast. A 1993 study involving more than 35,000 women aged 55-69 without a history of cancer found a 68 percent reduction in the risk of colon cancer in women with the highest intakes of vitamin E, compared to those with the lowest intakes. Results of the ATBC study showed that vitamin E supplementation reduced the incidence of prostate cancer by 32 percent and the risk of death due to prostate cancer by 41 percent.

High intake of vitamin C has been shown to provide protection against the development of certain cancers including those of the mouth, cervix, stomach, rectum, breast, lungs and prostate. A study involving more than 3,300 men and women found a 60 percent lower risk of colon cancer in those with the highest intake of vitamin C. A second study published in the *Journal of the National Cancer Institute* found women with the highest intake of vitamin C had a reduced risk of dying from breast cancer when compared to women with low vitamin

C intakes. A high intake of vitamin C is also associated with a reduced incidence of stomach cancer. Much of the evidence supporting the use of vitamin C in the prevention and/or treatment of cancer is based on a high dietary intake of the vitamin and not the use of supplements.

Antioxidants and Immunity

Evidence suggests that boosting immune function with antioxidants results in greater protection against acute infections as well as chronic disease, such as cancer, throughout one's life.

Vitamin C improves the response and function of white blood cells. Deficiencies in vitamin E can lead to significant impairments in immune function. A 1997 study reported in the *Journal of the American Medical Association* found a 4-6-fold improvement in immune function in a group of healthy subjects at least 65 years of age after only four months of supplementation with vitamin E (200 mg/day).

A selenium deficiency can increase a person's susceptibility to infections, while selenium supplementation has been shown to stimulate immunity by improving the function of white blood cells. Selenium supplementation can even help improve immune function in people with normal selenium concentrations in the blood. In one study, a daily dose of 200 mcg of selenium resulted in a 118 percent increase in the ability of lymphocytes (white blood cells) to kill tumor cells, and an 82 percent increase in the activity of natural killer cells. Avoid doses in excess of 400 mcg as they can be toxic.

Antioxidants and Diabetes

Increasing antioxidant status is vital in the prevention of long-term diabetic complications. Studies show that diabetics tend to have lower concentrations of antioxidants (in their blood) than non-diabetics. If you currently suffer from, or are at high risk for Type 2 diabetes, increase your dietary intake of antioxidants, especially vitamins E and C.

Antioxidants and Premature Aging

As you age, the level of free radicals in your system continues to increase, while the concentration of antioxidants most important to your health and well-being continues to fall.

A group of Italian researchers compared the amount of free radical damage and antioxidant levels in people over 100, with subjects 70-99 years of age. In the study, involving 82 individuals, researchers discovered that subjects over 100 had less free radical damage (as measured by lipid oxidation), and higher plasma levels of the antioxidants vitamin C and vitamin E, compared to the group aged 70-99. The results indicate that supplementation of antioxidants may help prevent premature aging.

While researchers noted high antioxidant levels in this study, it is important to understand that there is no evidence at this time showing that antioxidant supplements or antioxidant-enriched skin care products can help slow or reverse the aging process. Your best defense is to simply increase your dietary intake of antioxidants by eating more fresh fruits and vegetables and using a sunscreen with a minimum SPF rating of 15.

Antioxidants and Mental Decline

What's the most frightening aspect of growing old? For most of us it's the fear of senility. Dementia, one of the earliest signs of age-related mental deterioration, will afflict more than 20 percent of all Americans at some point in their lives. Several studies implicate free radical damage in brain aging and certain degenerative conditions associated with aging, including Alzheimer's disease. Researchers are examining the relationship between antioxidant status and mental health, as well as the effects of antioxidant supplements on the occurrence and various forms of dementia.

Data from the Nurses' Health Study, involving close to 15,000 former nurses ages 70-79 years, showed that women who had taken vitamin E and C supplements for several years performed better on a cognitive function test than women who had never taken the supplements. Longer use of the supplements was associated with greater benefit. Women who took only vitamin C derived no benefit.

A study published in the 2004 edition of the *Archives of Neurology* also provides convincing evidence of the benefit of antioxidant vitamins in the prevention of Alzheimer's. More than 5,000 men and women age 65 and over enrolled in the study. Subjects taking a combination of daily vitamin E (400 IU) and vitamin C (500 mg) supplements had a 4-5 times lower risk of developing Alzheimer's than subjects who did not take the combination of supplements.

B-Complex Vitamins

The production of energy in the body requires B complex vitamins. Vitamins B6, B12 and folic acid are essential for normalizing homocysteine levels in the blood. Homocysteine is an amino acid produced in the body, usually as a breakdown product of dietary protein. Elevated levels of homocysteine in the blood are associated with an increased risk for atherosclerosis, heart disease, stroke and Alzheimer's disease.

In the body, homocysteine is normally broken down into harmless byproducts with the help of vitamins B6, B12 and folic acid. Reduced intake of these B vitamins can lead to an unhealthy buildup of homocysteine in the blood. The consumption of B vitamin supplements helps normalize your homocysteine levels, and in turn, may help reduce your risk for cardiovascular and Alzheimer's disease.

B-vitamins are also essential for protein, carbohydrate and red blood cell metabolism, and normal functioning of the nervous and immune systems. Vitamin B6 deficiency depresses certain immune responses, whereas supplementation improves immune function. Vitamin B12 deficiency has also been linked to poor immune function, and B12 therapy has improved immune efficiency in B12 deficient individuals.

Ideally, choose a B-complex supplement that contains 400-1,000 mcg of folic acid, 10-50 mg of vitamin B6 and 50-300 mcg of vitamin B12. Some individuals may require up to 800 micrograms daily of folic acid to significantly reduce their homocysteine levels. Avoiding cigarettes and coffee may also help lower homocysteine levels in the blood. Vitamin B12 supplementation is especially essential for those following vegetarian diets, as a long-term deficiency can lead to irreversible brain damage.

Omega-3 Essential Fatty Acids

Of all the supplements discussed in this section, omega-3 fatty acids are by far the most important. Omega-3 fatty acids are crucial for good health and longevity. Several thousand scientific studies have demonstrated a wide range of conditions associated with omega-3 deficiencies, including heart disease, stroke, cancer, diabetes, arthritis, depression, inflammatory conditions and autoimmune disorders, allergies, ADHD symptoms, memory problems, and hair, skin and nail conditions.

Estimates indicate that close to 60 percent of the population is deficient in omega-3s. Most Americans consume excessive amounts of omega-6 fatty acids (from vegetable oils) and not nearly enough omega-3s (from fatty fish, ground flaxseeds and walnuts). Most research indicates that a proper balance of omega-3s and omega-6s is required for optimal health. The ideal ratio of omega-6 to omega-3 fats is 2:1. The average American's ratio of omega-6 to omega-3 is closer to 10:1, which spells trouble. This imbalance can increase the risk for many diseases.

In order to properly balance this ratio, you must increase intake of omega-3s while decreasing that of omega-6s. This is best accomplished by avoiding or limiting your intake of fried foods, processed foods, baked goods, and omega-6 rich oils, while increasing your intake of omega-3s through fish oil supplements. You can gain even more benefit by replacing oils high in omega-6s with those rich in a third type of fatty acid known as omega-9. Olive oil is monounsaturated, rich in omega-9s, and offers additional protection from heart disease by increasing good cholesterol.

Omega-3s and Heart Disease

Controlled clinical trials confirm that a steady diet of fish or fish-oil supplements plays a prominent role in the prevention of CHD. Omega-3s benefit the cardiovascular system because they lower triglyceride levels, reduce the formation of blood clots, fight inflammation within blood vessels, prevent heart arrhythmias, and improve the functioning of cells that line the heart and blood vessels. New research also suggests that fish oil can slow the progression of atherosclerosis, the buildup of plaque within arteries, when consumed at least once a week. This translates to a reduced risk of heart attack and stroke.

Results from the Nurses' Health Study found that women with the highest intake of omega-3s had about half the risk for CHD of those in the group with the lowest intake. In a 3 ½ year trial involving more than 11,000 heart-attack survivors, researchers found that survivors in the group given 1 gram of fish oil supplements daily had 20 percent fewer deaths overall, and 45 percent fewer sudden-death heart attacks than the untreated control group.

Omega-3s and Mental Function

A diet rich in the omega-3 fatty acid DHA also helps protect against memory loss and even slows or lowers the risk of Alzheimer's disease. Alzheimer's disease causes damage to synapses, the chemical connections between brain cells that enable learning and memory. DHA also protects against the synaptic damage and memory loss associated with this devastating illness. The brain absorbs DHA quickly, making a constant supply critical for proper cognitive function and mental tasks.

Omega-3s and Stress

Omega-3s help limit the damaging effects of stress. When Swiss researchers fortified men's diets with omega-3 fatty acids, levels of the stress hormone cortisol remained unchanged during stress tests, while the placebo group's cortisol levels rose by one-third.

Fish Oil Supplements vs. Fresh Fish

The best way to obtain the healthy benefits of fish is through fish oil supplements, which are free of the toxic pollutants found in most varieties of fish. Fish oils directly supply two important omega-3 fatty acids: EPA (eicosapentaenoic acid), which is essential for cardiovascular health, and DHA (docosahexaenoic acid), which benefits the nervous system.

Some of the strongest evidence supporting the use of fish oil supplements is at doses of 2 to 4 grams daily of EPA and DHA. This is also the dose currently recommended by the American Heart Association (AHA) if used under a doctor's supervision. If you suffer from a serious medical condition or are taking blood thinners, speak to your doctor before taking fish oil supplements since they can decrease the blood's ability to clot.

I also advise against the use of cod liver oil as a source of omega-3s. Cod liver oil is also rich in vitamins A and D, which can be toxic if taken in excess. While flaxseed contains no DHA or EPA, it is a rich source of the fatty acid alpha-linolenic acid (ALA), which can be converted to EPA in the body. Unfortunately, the body can only convert about 15 percent of it to EPA, making it a poor substitute.

***Important: Patients with implantable heart defibrillators have been found to have an increased risk of heart-rhythm abnormalities if they take too much omega-3s. Speak to your doctor prior to supplementing your diet with fish oils if you suffer from a serious medical condition.

Calcium

According to the National Osteoporosis Foundation, only 20 percent of adult women consume adequate amounts of calcium on a daily basis. On average, the typical American consumes only about 600 mg of calcium daily, far short of the recommended 1,000-1,500 mg. Unhealthy lifestyle habits such as cigarette smoking, excessive alcohol intake and a diet high in salt, animal proteins and soft drinks can further reduce the amount of calcium absorbed by the body.

Inadequate calcium intake and absorption put you at serious risk for osteoporosis and fractures of the hip, wrist and spine. More than 24 percent of all people suffering a hip fracture die within a year of the fall and another 50 percent never return to their prior level of mobility or independence. Women are not the only ones at risk for osteoporosis and life threatening fractures. A decline in bone density also occurs in men as they age. In fact, after age 65, the rate of decline for men equals that of women. The protective effect of calcium likely works in men as well as women. For these reasons, I recommend that both men and women supplement their diets with calcium and vitamin D.

Calcium can also help reduce the risk for colon polyps and colorectal cancer. One study reported that patients taking 1,200 mg of calcium daily for four years had 36 percent fewer colon polyps even five years after the trial had ended. In another study, women taking more than 800 mg of calcium daily reduced their risk of colorectal cancer by as much as 46 percent.

In addition to supporting bone density and reducing the risk of colorectal cancer, calcium plays a crucial role in regulating muscle contraction and relaxation (including the heart), blood clotting, regulating the secretion of insulin and transmitting nerve impulses—which, incidentally, can zip along at up to 300 feet per second.

To be effective, a calcium supplement should also contain vitamin D. Vitamin D enhances the intestinal absorption of calcium by up to 67 percent and helps maintain normal levels of calcium and phosphorous in the blood. Vitamin D can be produced naturally in the body with exposure (5-10 minutes daily) to the sun.

Ideally, your calcium supplement should contain 400 to 800 IUs of vitamin D. It's also important to choose the right form of calcium. Your body absorbs calcium citrate better than calcium carbonate by about 25 percent, whether it is taken on an empty stomach or with meals.

You should also be sure that your calcium supplement contains magnesium. Magnesium is another mineral that is essential for healthy bones. It contributes to increased bone density and helps prevent the onset of osteoporosis. Most people do not get enough magnesium in their diets, especially if they eat large amounts of processed foods in which much of the magnesium is removed. Since magnesium works closely with calcium, it is important to have an appropriate ratio of both minerals in order for them to be effective.

A good rule of thumb is a 2:1 calcium-to-magnesium ratio. For example, if you take 1,000 mg of calcium, you should also take 500 mg of magnesium. As with calcium, chelated forms of magnesium are absorbed best by the body. Magnesium chelated with amino acids is probably the most absorbable form. The newly available salts of magnesium aspartate or citrate are also good choices. Less absorbable forms include magnesium bicarbonate, magnesium oxide and magnesium carbonate.

Co-Q10

Co-Q10 is a naturally occurring vitamin-like nutrient that also possesses antioxidant properties. As we age, our bodies lose the ability to produce adequate amounts of Co-Q10 from dietary sources. Co-Q10 deficiency commonly occurs in people taking statin drugs for high cholesterol. Statins can block the synthesis of Co-Q10 in the body, which may lead to sub-optimal levels of Co-Q10 in the blood, and predispose statin users to heart disease. If you are currently undergoing statin therapy, I recommend that you discuss CoQ-10 supplementation with your physician.

Benefits of Co-Q10 supplementation include improvements in cardiac arrhythmias, reduced blood pressure, reduced damage to the heart following a heart attack, and increased tolerance for exercise. Co-Q10 is currently the most commonly prescribed treatment by physicians for congestive heart failure in Japan.

Garlic

Numerous studies have investigated the role and benefits of garlic supplements in preventing heart disease. Many of these studies showed positive benefits of garlic in heart disease: in particular, improving cholesterol profile. A few smaller studies have also suggested that garlic can reduce the incidence of blood clots and help bring down blood pressure.

Garlic can also help protect against certain cancers. The evidence is particularly strong for a link between garlic and prevention of prostate and stomach cancers. A large-scale epidemiological Iowa Women's Health Study examined the garlic consumption in 41,000 middle-aged women. Results showed that women who regularly consumed garlic had a 35 percent lower risk of developing colon cancer. Garlic contains sulfur and other compounds that slow or prevent the growth of tumor cells.

Unfortunately, to derive its health benefits, you would have to eat enormous quantities of garlic daily. The most efficient way of getting adequate and standardized amounts is by taking a nutritional supplement of garlic extract. I highly recommend using Kwai garlic, made from 100 percent organically grown Chinese garlic cloves, and standardized to ensure an effective and consistent level of allicin, the compound responsible for the cardiovascular benefits of garlic.

But allicin is not found in garlic. It's actually produced when garlic is crushed or digested. This is why taking a garlic supplement is preferred over natural garlic. Kwai garlic tabs are also coated to help ensure that they are odorless and are digested and absorbed in the intestine and not the stomach. Avoid consuming hot beverages with the tablets, since premature breakdown of the coating can occur.

Green Tea

A recent study presented at the 96th Annual Meeting of the American Association for Cancer Research 2005 found that green tea helps stave off prostate cancer. In the study, researchers looked at 62 men with precancerous prostate cells. Half of the men in the study were given a capsule containing 600 mg of green tea catechins daily (about 15 cups of green tea) and the other half were given a placebo (sugar pill). After one year, 30 percent of the men treated with the placebo developed prostate cancer while only 3 percent of the men taking the green tea capsules developed prostate cancer—a 90 percent reduction!

Green tea has also been shown to reduce many of the risk factors associated with heart disease, including elevated bad cholesterol and serum triglyceride levels, platelet aggregation and clot formation. Green tea protects against heart disease by reducing LDL cholesterol and triglyceride levels, increasing HDL levels, limiting oxidative damage to LDL cholesterol (responsible for the formation of plaques within the arterial wall) and inhibiting the formation of blood clots. Catechins found in green tea have also been found to inhibit the proliferation of smooth muscle cells lining blood vessels, a crucial process in atherosclerosis and cardiovascular disease.

In addition to cancer and heart disease, green tea has been found to benefit the following conditions:

- Diabetes—Significantly reduces oxidative damage to white blood cells.
- Stroke—Can reduce risk in nonsmoking women by 50 percent.
- Liver damage—Scientists at the University of North Carolina at Chapel Hill previously found that green tea extract increased the survival of fatty rat livers, damaged by alcohol exposure. They proposed that the extract could be used to help prevent liver transplant damage and failure.
- Viral infections—Catechins in green tea can inhibit enzymes required for the replication of HIV and herpes simplex virus.
- Bone strength—Men and women who regularly drank tea for more than 10 years were found to have higher bone mineral densities, even after exercise and calcium.
- Mood—Amino acids found in green tea have been shown to improve serotonin and dopamine levels in the brain.
- Rheumatoid arthritis—Antioxidants in green tea posses anti-inflammatory properties and may help prevent cartilage breakdown.

If you are concerned about wrinkles, age spots and other signs of aging, green tea may also help prevent or reverse the effects of aging. In animal studies, mice fed green tea demonstrated fewer signs of aging than those that were fed water.

Green tea can also help dieters lose weight. Catechins help with weight loss by improving the metabolism of carbohydrates, preventing fat deposition and promoting heat loss. To be effective, dieters should aim for 700 mg of catechins (green tea extract) daily.

In a recent study at Purdue University, researchers found that epigallocatechin gallate (EGCG), a compound found in the tea, inhibited the growth of cancer cells. The compound also killed cancer cells without causing harm to healthy tissue. This is one of the first studies to provide a direct link between epigallocatechin gallate and cancer inhibition. Green tea leaves are potent in EGCG. The study suggests that consumption of four to five cups of green tea may slow cancer. Previous studies have found a lower incidence of cancer in those who consume this amount of green tea, but the exact compound that produced this cancer inhibition is unknown.

Fiber

If you're not having regular bowel movements, I suggest adding an insoluble fiber supplement (25-35 grams daily) to your daily regimen. The extra fiber adds to the bulk of the stool and decreases the bowel transit time, which means better toxin elimination and better health. Keeping gut transit time to less than 20 hours seems to decrease the incidence of colon cancer.

Be sure to choose a fiber supplement that is rich in insoluble fiber (psyllium husk); the body does not absorb this type of fiber, so it passes through the bowel, carrying waste with it. Attempt to get 25-35 grams of fiber daily, whether from your diet, supplementation or a combination of the two. If you have never used a fiber supplement, be sure to increase your dose gradually; you may experience some initial stomach discomfort.

Aspirin Therapy

According to research published in the *Annals of Internal Medicine* (2002), taking a daily low-dose aspirin (75-150 mg) can reduce your risk of heart attack by approximately 30 percent. If you have already suffered a heart attack, taking aspirin can further slash your risk of a second heart attack by up to 50 percent. In addition, aspirin can also cut stroke risk in those who have had a previous stroke, and it reduces the risk of recurrent blockages in those who have undergone heart bypass surgery or other procedures such as angioplasty. Emerging research even suggests that aspirin can help prevent or reduce the risk of breast, prostate, ovarian and bowel cancers. Research has consistently found aspirin to be one of the most beneficial and most effective cardiac drugs available today when used properly.

So who should take aspirin? This issue is best discussed with your doctor, especially if you are a woman past menopause or a man over the age of 50. If you are younger, I recommend a daily aspirin only if you suffer from diabetes or two or more of the following criteria:

- Body weight that exceeds your ideal body weight by 30 percent or more
- Hypertension
- High cholesterol
- Smoking
- Family history of heart disease

As with all drugs, aspirin may cause adverse effects such as increased risk of bleeding in the digestive tract or brain, especially if you have uncontrolled high blood pressure, take anti-inflammatory drugs such as ibuprofen or take blood thinners. Also avoid aspirin if you suffer from an ulcer or consume more than three alcoholic beverages daily. It is highly recommended that you discuss the proper dose with your doctor, but new studies indicate that aspirin doses in the range of 75 to 150 mg are just as effective as 325 mg doses.

The Daily Essential Nutritional Supplements for Men and Women Include:

1. A daily multivitamin w/minerals (as directed on label)
2. Vitamin C (500 mg)
3. Vitamin E (400 IUs of mixed tocopherols)
4. Selenium (200 mcg)
5. B-complex vitamin (as directed on label)
6. Fish oil capsules (2-4 grams EPA and DHA)
7. Calcium citrate (800-1,200 mg) with added vitamin D (400 IUs) and magnesium (500 mg)
8. Garlic extract (Kwai; 300 mg 1-2 times)
9. Green tea extract (600 mg of catechins)

Optional

1. Co-Q10 (If you currently take a statin drug for high cholesterol or suffer from CHD) (100-150 mg)
2. Low-dose aspirin (75-150 mg) with your doctor's approval
3. Fiber supplement (25-35 grams)

In a Nutshell

If your goal is better health and an increased chance at longevity, then nutritional supplements make good sense. There are literally thousands of nutritional supplements from which to choose: lending to the confusion of what to take. The nutritional supplements recommended in this section are those I feel are most crucial to health and longevity. Their safety and effectiveness have been well-documented in the scientific literature and when combined with my eating plan and lifestyle recommendations, they can help significantly increase your chances of remaining healthy and living a long life.

One important concept to remember: Supplements are just what their name implies. They should play a supplemental or supporting role in your overall nutritional plan, whereas dietary sources should play the primary role. Nutritional supplements cannot negate damage caused by poor lifestyle habits such as eating nutrient-weak foods, not exercising, tobacco use and inadequate rest. If you currently suffer from a serious medical condition or other health concern, speak to your doctor before beginning nutritional supplementation.

Chapter 8 Goals

✓ Commit to a nutritional supplementation program featuring the supplements discussed in this chapter.
✓ Be sure to take nutritional supplements consistently or they will be of little value to your overall health and well being.

Chapter 9

Toxins—Hidden Dangers That Are Slowly Killing You

"The fact that the suburbanite is not instantly stricken has little meaning, for the toxins may sleep long in his body, to become manifest months or years later in an obscure disorder almost impossible to trace its origins."

~Rachel Carson

Life Extension Value: 2 Years

We are under assault. Our bodies have become the dumping grounds for thousands of toxins that invade our air, water, and food supplies. Worst of all, most people don't even realize what's happening to their bodies. These toxins build up slowly over time. We may not become acutely ill immediately after exposure to these substances so we suspect nothing. When our bodies reach the breaking point, the toxic build-up can lead to unexplained chronic conditions such as headaches, muscle aches and pains, constipation, sleeplessness, fatigue, gastrointestinal problems, anxiety, allergies, skin conditions, depressed immunity and other maladies that we fail to connect with this assault. If you don't want to end up a casualty of the war on your body, then you must educate yourself on the toxins in your environment and take action to limit your exposure and help your body rid itself of these dangerous intruders.

One study led by the Mount Sinai School of Medicine in New York at two major laboratories found an average of 91 industrial compounds, pollutants, and other chemicals in the blood and urine of nine volunteers, with a total of 167 chemicals found in the group. Of the 167 chemicals found, 76 are known to cause cancer in humans or animals, 94 are toxic to the brain and nervous system, and 79 cause birth defects or abnormal development. Other chemicals identified in the volunteers have been linked to cardiovascular and blood abnormalities, depressed immunity, abnormal changes in hormone levels, reproductive disorders, respiratory disorders, and digestive disorders, to name just a few.

It is estimated that the average person has between 400 and 800 chemical residues stored in the fat cells of their body. As these toxic compounds accumulate in our bodies, so too does their potential to make us sick. In fact, accumulation of toxic compounds in the body may be the most overlooked issue in healthcare today.

More evidence of this toxic war comes from the prevalence of cancer and cardiovascular disease, two of the main toxicity-related diseases. Columbia University School of Public Health reports that 95 percent of all cancers are caused by diet and environmental toxicity. A study appearing in the *British Medical Journal* (2004) estimates that perhaps 75 percent of most cancers are caused by environmental and lifestyle factors, including exposure to chemicals.

If you suffer from frequent, unexplained headaches, back or joint pain, tight or stiff neck, arthritis, chronic respiratory or sinus problems, asthma, abnormal body odor, bad breath, coated tongue, food allergies, poor digestion, chronic constipation with intestinal bloating or gas, brittle nails and hair, psoriasis, adult acne, unexplained weight gain over 10 pounds, unusually poor memory, chronic insomnia, anxiety, depression, irritability, chronic fatigue, or environmental sensitivities, especially to odors it's very likely that you're battling toxicity without even realizing it.

Because toxic compounds tend to accumulate in different parts of our bodies, at different rates, and in different combinations, they can cause a large variety of chronic illnesses and diseases. Early warning signs of toxic overload may include headaches and migraines, allergies, skin conditions, inflammatory and autoimmune diseases, chronic fatigue and more.

Would you ever purchase a high performance sports car and then fill it with cheap gasoline? If so, you probably wouldn't be surprised when your mechanic attributes your very costly repair bill to the use of cheap gasoline. Filling your body with these toxic impurities is no different. Eventually your performance will suffer and your body will break down. If you live an unhealthy lifestyle and believe that taking a few vitamins each day and going for a morning walk will do the trick, you're wrong. Optimal health has many components, all of which combine synergistically to help protect us from illness and disease. That's why the *Longevity Made Easy* plan involves multiple phases that work together as opposed to offering you a multiple choice approach to improving your health and wellness.

I'm not suggesting that you must live the remainder of your life inside a plastic bubble or survive on a diet of organic algae and distilled water as some authors would have you believe. I'm also not going to tell you to avoid every potential toxic compound that you might encounter such as cosmetics, toiletries, soap, shampoo, shaving creams, plastic wrap, and so on. For most people, this is an unreasonable solution.

What I am suggesting is a sensible and realistic approach toward limiting your exposure to common sources of toxins:

- Tobacco smoke and second-hand smoke
- Pesticides and herbicides
- Artificial sweeteners, preservatives and additives
- Processed and cured meats
- Drinking water
- Farm-raised salmon and large predator fish
- Unnecessary prescription and over-the-counter medications
- Trans fatty acids
- Alcohol
- Free radicals
- Stress

Avoiding or limiting your exposure to these toxins is a necessary step to help ensure continued health or to promote healing. The good news is that if you are having success thus far with the Synergy Plan then you have already reduced the amount of toxins assaulting your body. In addition to limiting exposure to these toxins, we must also find effective ways to eliminate some of the toxins already accumulated in our bodies. This phase of the Synergy Plan focuses on two main goals: eliminating and reducing exposure to common toxins and eliminating the toxins that have already accumulated in your body.

Meet the Toxins

Tobacco Smoke

To achieve optimal levels of health and increase your chances of longevity, if you are a smoker, you must stop. If you're currently a non-smoker, congratulations you have already increased your life expectancy by up to eight years! That's right, research shows that non-smokers live an average of six to eight years longer than smokers. Non-smokers should focus their efforts on avoiding or limiting their exposure to second-hand smoke.

Cigarette smoking is currently the most important preventable risk factor for heart disease and cancer, and is the leading cause of preventable death in America. Cigarette smoke contains more than 4,000 chemicals, including 200 known poisons. Harmful metals found in cigarette smoke include aluminum, copper, lead, and mercury. These deadly metals are also harmful to non-smokers as they are released into the environment as second-hand smoke. Non-smokers who work in smoke-filled environments may be just as much at risk as smokers for many of the diseases and conditions linked to smoking.

Smokers, the next time you feel the need to relax with a cigarette, why not enjoy a mixture of benzene and formaldehyde (available at your local funeral home as it is commonly used to preserve dead bodies), kitchen and bathroom cleaners, and exhaust fumes from your vehicle. Ah, that sounds nice and…deadly, doesn't it? That's in essence what each puff of your cigarette delivers. When you inhale these deadly poisons, your lungs absorb them and then transport them throughout your body causing extensive damage to nearly all tissues. Cigarette smoke causes permanent damage to the lungs, even in people who have only smoked a pack a day for one year. Cigarette smoke also contains high levels of endotoxin, the same poison produced by bacteria responsible for toxic shock syndrome and bronchitis. It's no wonder so many smokers complain of frequent bouts of respiratory infections and other ailments exacerbated by tobacco smoke such as asthma and allergies.

Here are more reasons to quit smoking. Smoking has been linked to the following conditions and diseases. Is that next cigarette really worth any of these?

- Heart disease, heart attacks, sudden cardiac death, angina, and irregular heart beats
- Strokes, blood clots, and brain hemorrhages
- Aortic aneurysm
- Increased risk of Type 2 diabetes
- Bronchitis, emphysema, pneumonia, and asthma
- Cancers of the lung, larynx, esophagus, stomach, bladder, liver, pancreas, kidney, mouth, prostate gland, and cervix
- Leukemia
- Gastritis and ulcers
- Anemia
- Impotence
- Osteoporosis
- Shortness of breath and fatigue
- Premature wrinkling
- Tooth loss, tooth discoloration, and gum disease
- Depression
- Infertility in men

As you can see, the illnesses and diseases linked to smoking are numerous and sometimes severe. Chances are, if you're a smoker, you'll suffer from a number of these conditions at some point in your life and will die prematurely as a result. According to the book The Costs of Poor Health Habits, each pack of cigarettes smoked costs the average smoker about 137 minutes of life expectancy. That may not seem like much, but over a lifetime, that can amount to a loss of six to eight years of life, not to mention a much poorer quality of life. Even smoking as little as one cigarette per day increases your risk of a heart attack by 40 percent. If you currently take aspirin or cholesterol lowering medications to protect your heart, smoking just three cigarettes a day wipes out the protective effects of these measures.

Gender, Age and Smoking

Smoking harms men, women, and children. For men, smoking is the number one cause of death by cancer. The average male smoker dies up to eight years sooner than men who do not smoke. Smoking also increases the risk of erectile dysfunction in men in their 30s and 40s by about 50 percent. Women don't fare much better. Female smokers age 35 and older die from chronic lung diseases such as bronchitis and emphysema more than 10 times as often as those who have never smoked. Lung cancer caused by smoking kills more women in the United States each year than breast cancer.

Secondhand Smoke

Nonsmokers who are exposed to secondhand smoke absorb nicotine and other compounds just as smokers do. In the U.S. alone, secondhand smoke is responsible for an estimated 35,000 to 40,000 deaths from heart disease and about 3,000 in cancer deaths in people who are not current smokers.

The 2006 US Surgeon General's report reached the following conclusions:

- Secondhand smoke causes premature death and disease in children and adults who do not smoke.

- Children exposed to secondhand smoke are at an increased risk of sudden infant death syndrome (SIDS), acute respiratory infections, ear problems, more severe asthma, and reduced lung growth.

- Exposure of adults to secondhand smoke has immediate and adverse effects on the cardiovascular system and causes coronary heart disease and lung cancer.

- The scientific evidence indicates that there is no risk-free level of exposure to secondhand smoke.

Tens of thousands of nonsmokers die in this country each year as a result of exposure to secondhand smoke. It is estimated that more than 126 million nonsmokers in the United States continue to be exposed to secondhand smoke. Smokers continue to claim that they have a right to smoke. They do not have a right to expose innocent people to deadly toxins and increase their risk for illness and death. Do your health a favor, and avoid exposure to secondhand smoke at all costs. Your life depends on it!

Kicking the Habit

Each year an estimated 1.5 million people in the U.S. successfully kick the habit, citing health concerns as the number one reason. Smoking cessation has major and immediate health benefits for smokers of all ages. Once you have stopped smoking for only one year, you reduce the excess risk of heart disease caused by smoking by nearly 50 percent. After 10 years of quitting, you reduce your risk of cancer by less than one-half that of those who continue to smoke. In 5-15 years, the risk of stroke for former smokers returns to the level of those who never smoked. Research has proved that smoking cessation, even in middle age, can substantially increase life expectancy. No matter your age or how long you've been smoking, you can still derive major health benefits from stopping now. It's never too late to quit.

Here's more motivation. Smoking cessation delivers these benefits and more:

- Increased life expectancy by up to 8 years
- Reduced risk of heart disease, stroke, cancer, and lung disease
- Reduced incidence of respiratory infections and allergies
- Increased energy levels
- Improved appearance of the skin and teeth
- Improved sense of smell and taste

So what is the best strategy to quit smoking? Studies have found that people are far more likely to kick the habit if they quit "cold turkey" than if they gradually cut back. On average, only about 10-12 percent of people actually succeed at quitting without any assistance. Using one of the smoking cessation aids on the market today can actually double your chances of success. Products that are currently available include antidepressants and nicotine patches, inhalers, nasal sprays, and gum/lozenges. These products are most effective if you truly have the desire to quit. Speak to your doctor about the benefits of each.

Here are a few strategies to help you quit smoking

- Make a commitment to quit smoking by setting a quit date, ideally a few weeks from today. Too much farther out and you may never get around to it.

■   Inform family members, friends, and co-workers that you have made a decision to quit smoking and ask for their understanding and support.

■   Encourage housemates, family members, or friends who smoke to quit with you or to avoid smoking in your presence.

■   Continue the exercise program from Phase Three. Smokers who exercise are more likely to succeed at quitting and are less likely to gain weight than smokers who do not work out. Physical activity is also associated with a greater life expectancy in smokers.

■   Anticipate the challenges of smoking cessation such as nicotine withdrawal, negative mood/depression, and the possibility of weight gain during the initial few weeks.

■   Remove all tobacco products from your home, office, and car including cigarettes, ashtrays, and lighters.

■   Make a list of all your reasons for quitting and repeat them several times daily.

■   If necessary, speak to your doctor about the use of nicotine-replacement products which can help to double your chances of success.

■   Join a support group in your area. A variety of organizations including the American Cancer Society, the American Lung Association (1-800-LUNG-USA), and the American Heart Association offer support programs to encourage and help people quit smoking.

Making the other changes described in this book will do little to improve your chances of health and longevity if you continue to smoke or expose yourself to second-hand smoke. Even one cigarette a day is too much. Make a commitment today to quit smoking and change your life forever. If you are a non-smoker you must eliminate your exposure to second-hand smoke. Do not frequent businesses and locations where you are likely to encounter second-hand smoke. In some cases, you may need to make changes at your work or home to avoid exposure to second-hand smoke.

Pesticides and Herbicides

We've already discussed in Chapter 4 the importance of choosing organic produce over conventionally grown fruits and vegetables. If you are still consuming non-organic produce, I want to provide you additional motivation to switch to organic. Consider that each year traditional farmers and growers spray their crops with more than one billion pounds of pesticides and herbicides in order to minimize losses. Estimates indicate that our food supply includes over 3,000 added chemicals and processed foods include more than 10,000 chemical solvents, emulsifiers, and preservatives.

Studies have found pesticide residues in up to 90 percent of the food we consume. Many of the pesticides in use today are carcinogenic, or cancer-causing. Others cause irreversible damage to the reproductive system, brain, and nervous system and compromise immunity. According to the World Health Organization (WHO), many commonly used pesticides could be a cause of cancer, birth defects, immune dysfunction, neurological illness, and sterility. Short-term effects of pesticide exposure include visual disturbances, nausea, vomiting, GI disturbances, tremors, and nerve damage. Farmers who use these chemicals on a daily basis have been found to be at an increased risk for certain cancers including cancer of the stomach, prostate, brain, and skin, as well as lymphomas and leukemia.

Pesticides do not belong in a healthful diet and should be avoided whenever possible. Always purchase organic produce and products when possible. Extensive testing carried out by the U.S. Department of Agriculture (USDA) shows that conventional fresh fruits and vegetables contain pesticide residues at levels three to 10 times higher, on average, than corresponding residues in organic samples. By consuming organically grown fruits and vegetables, you will virtually eliminate dietary exposure to dangerous pesticides and in the process, reduce the frequency and magnitude of one risk factor that can contribute to a variety of illnesses and diseases. The most heavily contaminated conventionally grown fruits and vegetables include apples, pears, peaches, nectarines, strawberries, cherries, celery, spinach and bell peppers.

Most supermarkets now offer a wide selection of organic produce and other products. It does cost a bit more, but the long-term health benefits are worth it. Don't think of it as an added expense today, think of it as a major source of savings later when your body rewards you with good health helping you keep down medical costs.

Artificial Sweeteners

Artificial sweeteners are commonly found in diet products, nutritional supplements, candies, desserts, and tabletop sweeteners. Of all the artificial sweeteners on the market today, aspartame (NutraSweet™) is by far the most dangerous. Long-term consumption of aspartame can have damaging neurotoxic, metabolic, and carcinogenic effects. It can take several years for these effects to occur, at which point the damage may be irreversible.

When consumed, aspartame breaks down into methanol which the body converts to formaldehyde, a potent nerve toxin and known cancer-causing agent used to preserve dead bodies. In his book, Health and Nutrition Secrets to Save Your Life, Dr. Russell Blaylock, a neurosurgeon and specialist in bioterrorism, states that it takes only one diet drink to cause significant DNA damage. Of approximately 100 independent studies conducted on aspartame, over 90 percent demonstrated significant health risks.

The consumption of products containing aspartame may lead to a wide array of health ailments including, but not limited to, the following:

- Brain tumors
- Birth defects
- Migraines and headaches
- Dizziness
- Depression and anxiety
- Seizures
- Visual disturbances
- Hearing loss and ringing in the ears
- Anxiety attacks
- Memory loss and confusion
- Slurred speech

- Joint pain
- Reduced sperm count

Aspartame can also worsen or mimic the symptoms of:

- Multiple sclerosis
- Fibromyalgia
- Arthritis
- Lupus
- Diabetes
- Depression
- Lymphoma
- Chronic fatigue syndrome
- Epilepsy
- Parkinson's
- Alzheimer's disease.

A study published in the *European Journal of Oncology* (2005) found that aspartame induces lymphomas and leukemia in rats at dose levels very near that to which humans can be exposed. In my opinion, aspartame should be immediately banned from all products. It is a highly toxic ingredient that has been clearly shown to be dangerous to humans. It only remains legal because the FDA wants to protect the profits of private industry rather than protect the public health. Of course since aspartame makes people sick, the drug industry wins as those people will need prescription drugs to mask the symptoms caused by aspartame. So, in effect, aspartame is a revenue generator for the pharmaceutical industry, and the FDA no doubt realizes this. More and more companies are now choosing alternative artificial sweeteners over aspartame for good reason.

Acesulfame-K is another popular artificial sweetener found in many diet and low-carbohydrate products. The safety of this sweetener is still in question as no significant studies have adequately tested it. The few studies involving acesulfame-K to date indicate that the sweetener causes cancer in animals. That means it could possibly increase the risk of cancer in humans as well. Again, limiting or avoiding the consumption of this artificial sweetener is your best option.

A third and very popular alternative sweetener is sucralose (Splenda™). Sucralose is produced by chlorinating sugar. Because it is made from sugar, it has been touted as a "natural" sweetener. This product is anything but natural. Animal studies have revealed that sucralose can cause a 40 percent shrinkage in the thymus gland (responsible for immune system function), swelling of the liver and kidneys, calcification of the kidneys, reduced growth rate, decreased red blood cell count, aborted pregnancy, and diarrhea among other things. Furthermore, no independent or long-term studies have yet evaluated the effects of sucralose in humans. The manufacturer claims that sucralose is safe because the body does not absorb it. These claims are false as the FDA's "Final Rule" report states humans absorb up to 27 percent of sucralose while the rest is excreted in the feces.

The reason most people give for consuming products containing artificial sweeteners is weight reduction. Here's something that will make it easier for you to stop ingesting these toxins: There are no studies to date showing that artificial sweeteners help people to lose weight. On the contrary, evidence exists indicating that artificial sweeteners may have the opposite effect. According to an article published in Technology Review, "Aspartame may actually stimulate appetite and bring on a craving for carbohydrates." In 1986, The American Cancer Society documented the fact that persons using artificial sweeteners gain more weight than those who avoid them and a Purdue University study comparing natural and artificial sweeteners found that animals fed artificial sweeteners ate more sugary foods.

Artificial sweeteners disrupt your body's natural ability to regulate appetite. In my opinion, the few calories you save by consuming artificial sweeteners are not worth the potential adverse heath risks associated with them. Be a smart consumer and start reading the labels on products you consume. As always, the closer to nature a product is, the healthier it tends to be. Optimal health is not created in the laboratory.

Rid your household of all products containing artificial sweeteners. Your body will thank you for it through better health. When it comes to sweeteners, it's best to stick with natural products such as unprocessed sugar, honey, or the herbal sweetener stevia. When used in moderation, natural sweeteners pose no harm and do not contribute to weight gain or abnormal spikes in blood sugar.

Processed and Cured Meats

Probably one of the worst choices you can make when it comes to animal products is processed lunch meats found at your local deli or supermarket. You should avoid these meats at all cost! Most of these products are highly processed with added chemicals and preservatives and are very high in sodium. Some of the preservatives contained in these products have been linked to stomach cancer. Many markets now offer healthier alternatives such as minimally processed and low-sodium varieties of lunch meat. Opt for these healthier selections whenever possible.

Research suggests that consumption of red and processed meats such as salami, sausage, scrapple, bacon, cured ham, hot dogs, and lunch meats can significantly increase an individual's risk of heart disease, stroke, colon cancer, and most recently, Type 2 diabetes. A study published in the November 2004 edition of the *Archives of Internal Medicine* found that the more red and processed meats people consumed, the higher their risk of diabetes rose. Having an additional serving of red meat daily increased the risk for diabetes by 26 percent, while adding another serving raised the risk by 40 percent.

Results of an ongoing study presented at the 2004 European Conference on Nutrition and Cancer further stress the importance of dietary choices and preparation methods. The study, involving almost half a million people from southern Greece to Norway, suggests that consuming preserved meats such as salami, bacon, cured ham, and hot dogs may increase the risk of bowel cancer by 50 percent. A recent study examining the relationship between diet and pancreatic cancer among nearly 200,000 men and women found that those who ate more than 1.5 ounces of processed meat a day were about two-thirds more likely to develop pancreatic cancer than those who avoided foods like hot dogs and sausages.

Studies of children who consumed more than 12 hot dogs per month showed them to have nine times the normal risk of developing childhood leukemia. Many processed meats contain nitrites which are used as preservatives. During the cooking process, nitrites combine with amines present in meat and in the stomach to form cancer-causing N-nitroso compounds which have been associated with cancers of the mouth, bladder, esophagus, stomach, and brain.

If you plan to eat meat, stick with fresh meat (preferably free-range) and avoid most of the commercial brands of processed meat.

Drinking Water

Many people are under the false assumption that our public water supply is free of contaminants and safe for regular consumption. The truth is quite the contrary. The correlations between contaminated water and cancer, cardiovascular disease, learning disabilities, and respiratory illness are becoming stronger and clearer.

Tap water contains many harmful impurities such as fluorine, arsenic, lead, iron, copper, silver, radon, and other heavy metals, all of which occur naturally. Other contaminants such as pesticides, herbicides, fertilizers, asbestos, cyanides, and other industrial chemicals also have a tendency to find their way into tap water. And if that's not bad enough, water treatment facilities intentionally add even more chemicals including chlorine, phosphates, lime, and aluminum sulfate to our water supply to kill various bacteria, viruses, and pesticides. An article appearing in USA Today indicates that the average city water supply contains more than 500 chemicals.

The EPA sets maximum contaminant levels (MCLs) for a broad range of drinking water contaminants. Even if the levels of each contaminant fall within the so-called "allowable limits", the sum of all these contaminants poses a significant risk to your health, especially if you currently suffer from a compromised immune system. Scientists are now discovering that even municipal drinking water additives, like chlorine and fluoride, meant to protect us from contaminated water, are as insidious and dangerous to our bodies as more commonly known poisons like nitrate and arsenic. Chlorine in drinking water is currently a leading cause of bladder and rectal cancer and asthma. Health officials are now linking chlorine ingestion to breast cancer, as well.

If you are wondering why these chemicals would be allowed in our water supply if they are so harmful, the answer is simple. We use a very small percentage of the public water supply for human consumption. We use most of the public water supply for things such as watering the lawn, doing laundry, washing cars, and taking showers. It would not be economically feasible to remove every chemical contained in the water supply for this reason. The public water authority is only concerned about contaminants that pose an immediate danger to humans.

Despite government regulations of drinking water, dangerous chemicals and other contaminants are constantly present in our tap water. Consuming clean water is an important component of overall health. Long-term consumption of unfiltered tap water can lead to health problems. Become most of us do not have access to pure glacier water, our next best choice becomes purified tap or bottled water.

Estimates indicate that about 25 percent of the bottled waters consumed in the U.S. come from municipal water supplies. Most go through significant processing such as reverse osmosis, deionization, activated carbon filtration, and other treatments. Of the water types listed, your best bet is probably purified water. Although it's likely from a municipal water supply, purified water has been treated extensively to remove many of the contaminants that are harmful to your health. Other types of bottled water may not have been treated as extensively and may not be any safer for consumption than tap water.

Be sure to purchase your bottled water in clear plastic or glass containers. Cheaper plastics like PVC (opaque one-gallon containers) have the ability to transfer toxins from the plastic such as methyl chloride into the water and contaminate it. I also advise against the consumption of distilled water as long-term consumption of distilled water can contribute to mineral deficiencies in the body and a slightly acidic PH, and may also be a factor in hypertension and cardiovascular disease.

If the thought of having to purchase bottled water from the store and transport it home seems like a burden, then a home water filtration system may be your best option. These systems are very economical and convenient, and are capable of producing high quality water. You can purchase a standard water filtration system at Home Depot or Lowes. If you do not have room for one of these systems or cannot afford one, Consumer Reports recommends the Culligan Filter as a better choice than Britta filters. Culligan Filters simply screw directly into your current faucet and are relatively inexpensive. You can check Consumer Reports online for additional recommendations if need be.

Farm-Raised Salmon and Large Predator Fish

We've already discussed the benefit of certain types of fish in your diet. We've also talked about the unhealthy level of contamination in most fish. True, salmon is rich in omega-3 fatty acids which are wonderful for the cardiovascular system and can help prevent or improve a myriad of conditions. Remember, however, that farm-raised salmon (the type served in most restaurants and found in supermarkets) contains very high levels of PCBs that can accumulate in our bodies and potentially increase our risk for cancer, liver disease, and other illnesses and conditions.

In January 2004, the journal *Science* warned that farmed salmon contains 10 times more toxins (PCBs and dioxin, among others) than wild salmon. The study recommends that farmed salmon be eaten no more than once a month and possibly only once every two months as they pose cancer risks to human beings. In July 2003, the Environmental Working Group (EWG) released a report stating that farmed salmon purchased in the United States contained the highest level of PCBs in the food supply system. In the report, EWG reported that farmed salmon have 16 times the amount of PCBs found in wild salmon. The EWG recommends that consumers choose wild instead of farmed salmon, and limit their intake of farmed salmon to less than 8 ounces once a month.

Mercury contamination of fish is fast becoming another serious health concern. In one of the nation's most comprehensive studies of mercury in commercial fish, testing by the Chicago Tribune found that a variety of popular seafood was so tainted that federal regulators could confiscate the fish for violating food safety rules. The Tribune's investigation reveals a decades-long pattern of the U.S. government knowingly allowing millions of Americans to eat seafood with unsafe levels of mercury. The report claims that "regulators have repeatedly downplayed the hazards, failed to take basic steps to protect public health and misled consumers about the true dangers, documents and interviews show." The report goes on to state that "eating canned tuna—one of the nation's most popular foods—is far more hazardous than what the government and industry have led consumers to believe."

Mercury can damage the central nervous system of children, causing subtle delays in walking and talking as well as decreased attention span and memory. Adults can experience headaches, fatigue, numbness in the hands and feet, and a lack of concentration. Two major European studies suggest that men also face an increased risk of heart attacks with increased exposure to mercury. Mercury is so toxic that a teaspoon of the metal is enough to contaminate a small lake.

The species of fish found to contain the high concentrations of mercury are known as "predator" fish and include shark, swordfish and tuna. In fact, almost all fish contains some level of mercury, much of which ends up in our oceans, lakes and streams as a result of air pollution. Small or short-lived species, such as shrimp, crab, flounder and tilapia, generally have lower amounts of mercury. Wild salmon, which eat plankton and small fish, are also low in mercury.

For the reasons mentioned, I recommend avoiding or restricting your intake of all farmed and canned fish and shell fish. Enjoy the heart healthy benefits of fish by consuming wild salmon which has been found to contain much lower levels of PCBs and other toxins than their farm-raised counterparts. Wild Alaskan salmon eat Pacific Ocean fish that are naturally lower in persistent pollutants, and they carry less fat than farmed salmon. You can purchase wild Alaskan salmon at local fish markets and at a limited number of supermarkets. Most canned salmon is of the wild variety as well. You can also make the most of salmon's healthy benefits without exposing yourself to dangerous PCBs by taking fish oil supplements which have been found for the most part to be free of mercury and PCBs.

Unnecessary Prescription and Over-The-Counter Drugs

Blink too much? Smile too much? Scared to speak in public? Got sweaty palms? There's a drug that can help! But at what cost? There's no denying the fact that America has become an overmedicated society. For every complaint, there seems to be a drug, or a combination of drugs designed to treat it.

The side effects caused by many drugs are sometimes more severe than the conditions they are designed to treat. What most "pill poppers" fail to realize is that every drug, whether prescription or over the counter (OTC), has adverse effects that range from mild stomach upset to even death. According to estimates between 100,000 to 400,000 Americans die each year from adverse drug reactions and another 1,000,000 people require hospitalization due to adverse drug reactions. The leading causes of adverse drug reactions include antibiotics (17 percent), cardiovascular drugs (17 percent), chemotherapy (15 percent), and analgesics and anti-inflammatory agents (15 percent).

Contrary to popular belief, even NSAIDs such as aspirin, ibuprofen (Motrin, Advil), and naproxen (Aleve) are not safe. Studies estimate NSAID-related death in the United States at 10,000 to 20,000 per year, and NSAID-related hospitalizations at 100,000 per year. In fact, all medications, including OTC medications, are in one way or another, toxic to the body.

Since 1997, more than a dozen prescription drugs have been taken off the market due to serious side-effects. Many Americans continue to operate under the false assumption that because a drug has been approved by the FDA and prescribed by their doctor that it is safe to take. As Vioxx, Aleve and many other drugs have already proved, this is often not the case. Several other drugs have since been pulled from the market or contain new warnings due to the serious adverse reactions associated with their use.

Healthy individuals understand that health does not come in the form of a pill. Rather than addressing the cause of disease, most medications merely mask symptoms of illness and disease, giving an individual a false impression that they are, in fact, healthy. Here's the fact: if you are taking medication of any type, you are not healthy. If you were healthy, you would not require medication. Medical technology, diagnostic testing, overuse of medical and surgical procedures, and overuse of pharmaceutical drugs may actually be contributing to illness and disease.

When I suggest eliminating all unnecessary medications from your daily regimen I'm not referring to medications used to control a potentially dangerous medical condition such as high blood pressure, cholesterol, or diabetes. I'm talking about over-the-counter pain relievers and prescription medications that are commonly over-prescribed by doctors. Antibiotics are a good example of the type of medication to which I am referring. They continue to be one of the most over-prescribed medications. Studies indicate that more than 40 percent of about 50 million physicians' prescriptions for antibiotics each year are inappropriate. Even more disconcerting is when you consider that using antibiotics, when not needed, can lead to the development of deadly strains of bacteria that are resistant to drugs and cause more than 88,000 deaths per year due to hospital-acquired infections.

Elderly individuals are at highest risk for serious complications from medications due to the high number their doctors commonly prescribe. On average, these individuals take between 2-4 types of prescription medications daily, and the older they are the more they take. Studies have shown that the more doctors a patient has, the more drugs they will be taking, thus increasing the likelihood of dangerous interactions and serious complications.

Rather than being a passive recipient of whatever drug your physician prescribes to you or that has been advertised as "safe," take personal responsibility and work actively with your physician and your pharmacist. Make sure that you are only taking drugs that are absolutely necessary. Even for necessary drugs, a lower dosage may still be effective. Ask your doctor whether you can safely experiment with taking a reduced amount. Make sure you understand any risks and possible side-effects associated with the drugs you are taking—especially if they are prescribed for long-term use, or if you take multiple medications. You can check them out yourself in the Physicians' Desk Reference, available at most libraries. Newer drugs are not always better as they have a limited safety record. It's estimated that as many as 20 percent of newly-approved prescription drugs have unexpected adverse reactions. OTC drugs become part of your toxic load as well. Occasional use of an OTC remedy may have no ill effects, but be careful about long-term or repeated exposure to any chemical agents.

Remember that, just because your doctor prescribes a drug for you or because it's available to you without a prescription doesn't mean that it's not toxic to your body. All drugs are foreign to your body and should thus be treated as such. Work with your doctor to eliminate all unnecessary medications from your daily regimen. If you doctor is unwilling to work with you, then find one who is. Your health and life may depend on it. Many people have found alternative therapies or lifestyle changes that can eliminate or reduce the need for pills through consultation with an alternative medicine-oriented M.D. or naturopath physician.

Trans Fatty Acids

Trans-fats are, by far, the unhealthiest oils you can consume. Trans-fatty acids are worse for your cardiovascular system than saturated fats. While saturated fats only raise LDL cholesterol while leaving HDL cholesterol unaffected, trans-fatty acids contribute to cardiovascular disease by reducing HDL (good) cholesterol and increasing LDL (bad) cholesterol. According to some estimates, the consumption of trans fats causes up to 100,000 premature heart disease deaths each year. These "killer fats" interfere with the metabolism of beneficial omega-3 and omega-6 fatty acids and cause hormonal imbalances, interfere with cell membrane reproduction, and encourage the development of certain cancers. They have also been linked to diabetes and Alzheimer's disease.

You should avoid trans-fats at all cost. You can locate trans-fats in food products by carefully reviewing the labels. Products containing the words "hydrogenated," "partially hydrogenated", or "vegetable shortening" should not be consumed. Consider them lethal and keep them out of your pantry and out of your body. Most margarines, snack foods, baked goods, cookies, and convenience meals include hydrogenated vegetable oils. You'll also find these killer fats in many processed foods like prepared meals and nearly all fried foods. The FDA recently announced that beginning in 2006 food manufacturers will be required to list the amount of trans fats contained in their products. Fortunately, many companies are now taking steps to eliminate trans fats. Start reading product labels and avoid all foods containing trans fats or partially hydrogenated oils in their list of ingredients.

Alcohol

Moderate alcohol intake—one or two glasses of wine or beer daily—may be beneficial to the cardiovascular system and can even help to protect you from cardiovascular disease. Excessive intake of alcohol can lead to cirrhosis of the liver and its complications, including liver cancer. It has also been linked to an increased risk for colorectal and breast cancers, high blood pressure, gastrointestinal complications, such as gastritis and ulcers, overweight and obesity, and the depletion of certain vitamins and minerals. When it comes to alcohol, moderation is key.

Free Radicals

If you are successfully implementing my eating and nutritional supplementation plans then you are limiting your exposure to free radicals. You'll recall that free radicals are highly reactive, toxic substances that the body produces during normal functions such as respiration and metabolism. Because free radicals are missing an electron, they roam the body seeking electrons to steal from other molecules. Free radicals have been implicated in over sixty different health conditions including cardiovascular disease, cancer, diabetes, and premature aging. Free radicals have also been linked to the development of neuro-degenerative diseases such as Alzheimer's disease and Parkinson's disease.

Free radicals can result from:

- Environmental pollutants such as smog, heavy metals (mercury, cadmium and lead), radiation, tobacco smoke, herbicides, pesticides
- Sun exposure
- Over-the-counter medications
- Prescription drug interactions
- A high fat diet
- Regular exercise

Although you cannot completely avoid exposure to free radicals, you can take steps to minimize the amount of damage caused by them. If you are following the Synergy Plan then you are engaging one of the best defenses against free radicals: antioxidants. A diet rich in antioxidants helps neutralize the harmful effects of free radicals and has been shown to offer protection against heart disease, cancer, stroke, diabetic complications, cataracts, mental deterioration, and premature aging. The Synergy Eating Plan and nutritional recommendations ensure that you will have an adequate intake of antioxidants to combat the harmful effects of free radicals. You should also limit your exposure to the sun, tanning beds, conventionally grown produce and to foods high in fat.

Stress

Although very few people consider it as a toxin, stress can be highly toxic to the body. Chronic stress can precipitate a host of destructive processes including immune suppression, hypertension, muscle wasting, fatigue, impaired mental function, fluid retention, thinning of the skin, and even premature aging. Stress chemicals reduce blood supply to the skin and also slow down the body's normal repair processes, depriving the skin of needed nutrients and causing cells in the basal layer of the epidermis to divide more slowly. As a result, the skin doesn't renew itself as quickly and wounds don't heal as quickly; essentially the skin is "older".

Chronic exposure to stress, whether at home or at work, can also double your risk for a heart attack. People who have little control on the job or at home appear to be at highest risk for stress-related cardiovascular disease. Modern life is full of unavoidable external stressors, and the way we respond to these events is what matters. In fact, how you choose to respond to a stressful event makes all the difference, and new ways of responding can be learned.

You already know from Chapter 3 that many people find techniques such as breath control, meditation, and yoga helpful in keeping stress levels down on a daily basis. Stress causes the release of specific hormones in the body which over time can be toxic. Practicing the stress-reduction techniques outlined in Chapter 3 will help you develop effective coping mechanisms for stress. Keep in mind that to be effective, stress reduction techniques must be practiced regularly, especially during times of high stress.

Detoxification

One of the body's natural means of staying healthy is its ability to detoxify itself. Through detoxification, your body renders harmless and expels many of the dangerous compounds that it has absorbed, inhaled, or created. Detoxification is essentially the process of removing or neutralizing toxins in the body. The primary organs of detoxification are the bowels, liver, kidneys, lungs, and skin.

Following my *Longevity Made Easy* plan will greatly limit your exposure to deadly toxins, but you may still require a systematic plan for ridding your body of the toxic build-up from years past. Effective techniques for detoxification include chelation therapy, fasting, colonics, nutritional protocols, and body work. Literally thousands of books cover the principles of detoxification, so I'll avoid going into a lengthy detailed discussion on the topic. Instead I will provide a few simple and effective detox techniques.

Fasting Guidelines for Detoxification

Fasting is an excellent way to rid your body of toxic accumulation. You should undergo my simple fasting plan once to begin your detoxification program and repeat it every few months if possible. Here are the steps to my simple fast.

1.   Avoid the temptation to gorge yourself on junk food or other foods the night before your fast. Consume a light and healthy diet consisting primarily of fresh fruits and vegetables for several days prior to beginning your fast.

2.   Avoid consuming caffeine and alcohol during your fast as they can stress your body during the detoxification process. To avoid a caffeine withdrawal headache, you may want to wean yourself off of it a few days prior to beginning your fast. Bottled or purified water with added lemon or lime is the beverage of choice for most people while fasting.

3.   Be aware that you may experience headaches, nausea, jitters, diarrhea, and other symptoms as your body rids itself of toxins and begins to detoxify itself. If you have been eating an unhealthy diet for many years and have never fasted, these

symptoms may be more pronounced. This is actually a good sign that your body is "clearing" itself of unhealthy toxins.

4. Your fast can last anywhere from one to several days. If you have never fasted, I recommend beginning with a one day fast consisting of purified or bottled water with some added lemon or lime juice. You should attempt to drink up to one gallon of water daily to help assist your body in the removal of toxic waste. If needed, you may also consume a small amount of fresh organic vegetable juice (made in a juicer) during your fast. You can also try alternating water-fasting with juice-fasting if water-only fasting seems too difficult during extended fasting periods. For example, 1 day on organic vegetable juice, 1 day on water.

5. If a complete fast seems too difficult, consider a partial fast. A partial fast involves restricting yourself to a diet of clean water and fresh organic fruits and vegetables while avoiding meats, fish, dairy, and eggs. You can perform partial fasts for several days without difficulty.

6. Avoid strenuous activity during your fast as it places stress on your body interfering with your body's ability to detoxify itself. Walking and stretching can be of benefit during a fast as they can help to rid toxins from the lymphatic system. Saunas and steam rooms can also help with the elimination of toxins through the skin.

7. Continue to eat healthy and light for several days after your fast has ended. Avoid the temptation to eat starchy or sugary foods as they can undo many of the health benefits of your fast.

8. For continued health, try fasting once every few months, if possible. As your body becomes more accustomed to fasting, try increasing the length of your fasts and varying the forms of fasting.

9. Always check with your doctor prior to beginning a fast, especially if you suffer from any serious health concerns. Pregnant or breastfeeding women, individuals with heart problems, diabetes and who are underweight should not fast.

10. Long-term fasting—beyond three days—should only be done under medical supervision. You can locate a practitioner who specializes in therapeutic fasting through the International Association of Hygienic Physicians at http://www.iahp.net or by calling (330) 788-0526.

Nutritional Supplements That Support Detoxification

Take nutritional supplements that support the function of the liver, kidneys, gut, and skin. Two of the most important supplements may be milk thistle and fiber. Begin supplementation approximately one week prior to beginning your fast and continue supplementing for about one week after you have ended your fast.

Milk Thistle (250 mg standardized extract three times daily)

The liver, which is responsible for detoxifying pollutants and processing nutrients and fats, is the body's second largest organ. Milk thistle has been shown to protect and enhance the function of the liver. The German Commission E lists milk thistle as an approved herb for "toxic liver damage, inflammatory liver disease, and cirrhosis," with no side effects other than an occasional mild laxative action. Milk thistle strengthens liver cells and prevents toxins from harming the liver. It also boosts levels of glutathione, which is crucial to the liver's role in detoxification. Although there are better-known antioxidants, including vitamins A, C, and E and the mineral selenium, milk thistle is 10 times more potent in the liver. Milk thistle can also help promote the regeneration of new liver cells and alleviate a host of ailments associated with the liver, such as hepatitis and cirrhosis. Milk thistle also possesses the ability to reduce inflammation and possibly retard skin cell proliferation, a mechanism that can lead to such conditions as psoriasis. I recommend taking milk thistle several days prior to beginning your fast and continuing it for up to a week after it has ended.

Fiber

For fasts lasting more than a day, you may want to consider the use of a fiber supplement to help aid in the excretion of waste material from the gut. Frequent constipation can cause toxic compounds to accumulate in the bowel and over time leads to gastrointestinal disorders. If waste matter is not eliminated from the gut, toxic residue may be reabsorbed into the bloodstream and cause poor health and disease. Consume a teaspoon or two of fiber mixed with water each morning.

In a Nutshell

Our bodies are under attack. The environment we live in today fires thousands of toxins at us on a daily basis. The ultimate goal of any detoxification program should be to limit the intake of toxic compounds while stimulating the body to remove the ones that are presently stored in the body. For those who choose to follow a healthful diet rich in organic fruits and vegetables and live a healthy lifestyle the process of detoxification will come naturally.

For those who want the benefits of optimal health but don't want to make the sacrifices, it probably seems like too much to ask. Good health is within our reach, but to get there we must first put forth a consistent effort to live a healthy lifestyle and rely less on drugs and surgery. Too many people today have never known or have forgotten what it "feels" like to be healthy. They are depressed, stressed out, overmedicated, overweight, and struggling to find the energy to get through each day. If you are one of these people, it may be a good time to begin a detoxification program. In this chapter I have presented you with a simple plan and guidelines to begin the detoxification process.

I regularly engage in a 1-2 day fast consisting of clean water and a small amount of organic vegetable juice and feel wonderful afterwards. You can learn more about fasting and specific detoxification programs through numerous publications. Remember, to successfully detoxify your body you must also avoid or limit your exposure to the toxins that are present in our everyday lives and nourish your body with the food and nutritional supplements that can offer protection against these toxic compounds. With these simple, yet deliberate actions, you can slow the assault on your body and greatly improve your chances of a long and healthy life.

Chapter 9 Goals:

✓   Eliminate or reduce your exposure to as many of the toxins mentioned in this section as possible.
✓   Consume a healthful diet rich in organic fresh fruits and vegetables to promote natural detoxification.
✓   Consider a periodic 1-2 day fast consisting of clean water and a small amount of organic vegetable juice to help further rid your body of stored toxins.

Chapter 10

Life Saving Medical Tests You Can't Afford To Ignore

Following a routine physical exam that included the usual procedures such as blood tests and listening to the heartbeat, an apparently healthy 45-year-old man is given a "clean bill of health" by his physician. A few weeks later the man suffers a massive heart attack while walking and dies. His family, friends and even his doctor are stunned. The doctor blames family history of heart disease—despite the victim not having previously showed any obvious signs of cardiac problems. This happens often.

I was speaking with a former patient of mine one day at a coffee shop and was stunned to learn that her husband had passed away from a heart attack. She was in total shock because he had very good cholesterol levels. I explained that many people with normal cholesterol drop dead every day of heart attacks because an individual's risk for heart disease is based on much more than just cholesterol levels. Approximately half of all people who suffer heart attacks have a normal lipid profile (cholesterol, HDL, LDL, triglyceride level).

With visits to your doctor becoming shorter (average visit is now seven minutes) and seeing multiple providers who may not always be familiar with your health history, it's imperative that you take responsibility for your own health and well-being. It is not your doctor's job to "keep you healthy." That's your responsibility.

Most people see their doctor only when they are injured or feeling ill. Imagine calling your doctor's office to make an appointment for health and wellness. When the receptionist asks, "What's wrong?" you state, "Nothing," and proceed to explain that you want to make sure you are healthy. I can assure you that this happens rarely and would in most cases surprise the entire staff including the doctor himself.

Health-minded individuals take full responsibility for their health. They request pertinent medical tests and exams, and are not afraid to question their physician about test results or medications they have been prescribed. Many people actually cannot even name their various medications: "Oh, it's some long name, I can't recall," or, "Um, well, I can't think of the name of it."

Questioning your doctor doesn't mean you don't trust him or her. Yet many people will drill their car mechanic about exactly what's wrong with their car and exactly what's going to be done about it, but when it comes to their own body they suddenly become silent. Perhaps they are too afraid to ask. That is a big mistake.

Things can be missed during routine medical visits. Most doctors today simply don't have the time to sort through your entire medical history, review previous lab tests and results, track test values over time and follow up with you on the results of these tests. This is why it's essential that you keep a medical diary of all significant health-related events, including the doctors you have seen, specific tests that were ordered and the results of those tests, and any prescribed medications.

You should also document any major emotional and physical stresses and any unusual health symptoms you may have experienced since the previous visit. This will keep your health information organized, and in turn, help you get the most from each visit to your doctor.

If your doctor orders specific tests, always request a copy of the results for your records, even if your doctor insists they are normal or says he will call you only if there is something abnormal. According to the American College of Physicians' Code of Ethics, ethically and legally, you are entitled to the information in your records. If your doctor refuses to provide you with a copy of your medical records, it may be time to find another doctor.

With that said, there are certain tests that can actually save your life. Early detection and treatment is the key for many life-threatening illnesses and diseases, especially when it comes to heart disease and cancer. Because our risk for illness and disease tends to increase with age, I have included specific tests and the age when they should be ordered.

Your doctor or insurance company may not agree that you need or that you can benefit from these tests, but many do. If your insurance company refuses to cover a specific test, then pay for it yourself. The sad truth is most people have no problem paying out-of-pocket for cosmetic improvements, home improvements and automobile maintenance, but frown upon having to pay for a few simple and relatively inexpensive medical exams that could save or add years to their life.

Even those of us with access to the best medical care available can have undiagnosed disease. More aggressive use of preventive screening exams, such as blood marker tests and noninvasive scans, may help identify those most at risk for conditions such as heart disease and cancer and provide a better opportunity for early intervention, especially in high risk populations.

Cancer is a "silent killer." This is because many types of cancer have a slow, insidious onset without early symptoms. For this reason, regular screening for common types of cancer is valuable and can help save your life. If all Americans followed early detection recommendations set forth by the American Cancer Society (ACS), the 5-year survival rate for cancers of the skin, mouth, breast, colon, rectum, cervix, prostate and testes might be about 95 percent.

Heart disease and stroke are other silent killers that have a slow, secretive onset without early symptoms. As previously mentioned these conditions begin developing in our teens and can become progressively worse with age.

A few simple blood and imaging tests can help identify these diseases in their early stages and give you the best chance of treating and even reversing them before it's too late. Experts estimate that 90 percent of all strokes could be prevented if people at risk were identified and treated early enough.

Some of the tests listed below are on the cutting edge of medicine and are of still unproven value. They can be difficult to interpret and in some cases, offer false-positive results that lead to unnecessary treatments. Nonetheless, you should still discuss the benefits of these tests and exams with your doctor.

Keep this page bookmarked and check off every test that you've undergone with the date. You should also save a copy of the results for each test after reviewing the findings with your doctor. Remember, you are responsible for your health and well-being, not your physician.

Men 20—39 Years

Monthly
o Testicular self-exam
o Skin self-check for suspicious moles

Yearly
o Blood pressure check
o Clinical testicular exam
o Dilated eye exam (for diabetics)

Every 3 years
o Fasting lipid panel
o Fasting blood-glucose test
o Clinical skin exam

Every 5 years
o Routine physical exam

Variable
o HIV test (for sexually active individuals with multiple partners, or IV
   drug users)
o C-reactive protein (see test description and recommendation below)
o Homocysteine (see test description and recommendation below)
o Lipoprotein-A (see test description and recommendation below)
o EKG (one at age 35 to establish a baseline measure of heart function)

Immunizations
o Tetanus-diphtheria booster: every 10 years
o Hepatitis B vaccine: once, for at-risk people

Women 20—39 Years

Monthly
o Breast self-exam for abnormal lumps
o Skin self-check for suspicious moles

Yearly
o Blood pressure check
o Clinical breast exam
o Dilated eye exam (for diabetics)

Every 2 years
o TVU (for women with a moderate-to-strong family history of either ovarian or breast cancer)
o Digital mammogram (for women with a moderate-to-strong family history of ovarian or breast cancer)

Every 3 years
o Fasting lipid panel
o Fasting blood-glucose test
o Clinical skin exam
o PAP test and pelvic exam

Every 5 years
o Routine physical exam

Variable
o HIV test (for those at risk)
o C-reactive protein (see test description and recommendation below)
o Homocysteine (see test description and recommendation below)
o Lipoprotein-A (see test description and recommendation below)
o BRCA1 and BRCA2 (for those with a family history of breast or ovarian cancer)
o EKG (one at age 35 to establish a baseline measure of heart function)

Immunizations
o Tetanus-diphtheria booster: every 10 years
o Hepatitis B vaccine: once, for at-risk people

Men 40—49 Years

Monthly
o Testicular self-exam
o Skin self-check for suspicious moles

Yearly
o Blood pressure check
o Clinical testicular exam
o Digital rectal exam
o Dilated eye exam (for diabetics)

Every 3 years
o Routine physical exam
o Fasting lipid panel
o Fasting blood-glucose test
o Clinical skin exam

Variable
o HIV test (for those at risk)
o C-reactive protein (see test description and recommendation below)
o Homocysteine (see test description and recommendation below)
o Lipoprotein-A (see test description and recommendation below)
o Exercise stress test
o EBCT (every five years for men over 45 with traditional risk factors
  for heart disease)

Immunizations
o Tetanus-diphtheria booster: every 10 years
o Hepatitis B vaccine: once, for at-risk people

Women 40—49 Years

Monthly
o Breast self-exam
o Skin self-check for suspicious moles

Yearly
o Clinical skin exam
o Blood pressure check
o Clinical breast exam
o Dilated eye exam (for diabetics)

Every 2 years
o Digital mammogram (more accurate than a traditional mammogram
  for this age group)

Every 3 years
o Routine physical exam
o Fasting lipid panel
o Fasting blood-glucose test
o PAP test, pelvic exam and digital rectal exam

Variable
o HIV test (for those at risk)
o C-reactive protein (see test description and recommendation below)
o Homocysteine (see test description and recommendation below)
o Lipoprotein-A (see test description and recommendation below)
o Exercise stress test
o BRCA1 and BRCA2 (for those with a family history of breast or ovarian cancer)

Immunizations
o Tetanus-diphtheria booster: every 10 years
o Hepatitis B vaccine: once, for at-risk people

Men 50+ Years

Monthly
o Testicular self-exam
o Skin self-check for suspicious moles

Yearly
o Routine physical exam
o Blood pressure check
o Clinical testicular exam
o Fecal occult blood test
o PSA test
o Dilated eye exam (for diabetics)

Every 3 years
o Fasting lipid panel
o Fasting blood-glucose test
o Clinical skin exam
o Dilated eye exam

Every 3 to 5 years
o Thyroid-stimulating hormone (TSH) test

Every 5 years
o Spiral CT Scan (for moderate-to-heavy lifetime smokers)

Every 10 years
o Colonoscopy
o Abdominal ultrasound for AAA (if family history of aneurysm, smoker, people with HTN, CAD, or over age 65)

Variable
o HIV test (for those at risk)
o C-reactive protein (see test description and recommendation below)
o Homocysteine (see test description and recommendation below)
o Lipoprotein-A (see test description and recommendation below)
o Exercise stress test
o EBCT (every five years for men with traditional risk factors for heart disease)
o Duplex ultrasound of the carotid arteries (for people who have experienced TIAs or mini-strokes)

Immunizations
o Tetanus-diphtheria booster: every 10 years
o Hepatitis B vaccine: once, for at-risk people
o Influenza vaccine: every year if 65 or older or with chronic disease
o Pneumovax: every six years beginning at 65 or if you suffer from chronic disease

Women 50+ Years

Monthly
o Breast self-exam
o Skin self-check for suspicious moles

Yearly
o Routine physical exam
o Blood pressure check
o Clinical breast exam
o Clinical skin exam
o Mammogram
o Digital rectal exam
o Fecal occult blood test
o Dilated eye exam (for diabetics)

Every 3 years
o Fasting lipid panel
o Fasting blood-glucose test
o PAP test and pelvic exam (may discontinue at age 65 if all tests were
   normal)
o Dilated eye exam

Every 3 to 5 years
o Thyroid-stimulating hormone (TSH) test

Every 5 years
o Spiral CT Scan (for moderate-to-heavy lifetime smokers)

Every 10 years
o Colonoscopy
o Abdominal ultrasound for AAA (if family history of aneurysm,
   smoker, people with HTN, CAD, or over age 65)

Variable
o HIV test (for those at risk)
o C-reactive protein (see test description and recommendation below)
o Homocysteine (see test description and recommendation below)
o Lipoprotein-A (see test description and recommendation below)
o Exercise stress test
o EBCT (every five years for women over 55 with traditional risk factors for heart disease)
o Duplex ultrasound of the carotid arteries (for people who have experienced TIAs or mini-strokes)
o Bone mineral density test (after menopause)

Immunizations
o Tetanus-diphtheria booster: every 10 years
o Hepatitis B vaccine: once, for at-risk people
o Influenza vaccine: every year if 65 or older or with chronic disease
o Pneumovax: every six years beginning at 65 or if you suffer from
   chronic disease

Test Descriptions

Cardiovascular Disease

The following tests can help detect the disease during its early stage when it's most treatable, and may reduce the need for aggressive and risky procedures.

Lipid Panel

A lipid panel measures the fats (lipids) in your blood. The measurements can indicate your risk of having a heart attack, stroke or other cardiovascular disease. It typically includes the following:

- LDL cholesterol, the "bad" cholesterol
- HDL cholesterol, the "good" cholesterol
- Triglycerides
- Total cholesterol—the sum of your blood's HDL cholesterol and a portion of triglycerides

CRP (C-reactive protein)

CRP is a protein found in the blood that your liver produces as part of your immune system's response to injury or infection. It's also produced by muscle cells within the coronary arteries. CRP is a nonspecific sign of inflammation, which means it may not be clear what's causing the inflammation.

High levels of CRP in your blood are associated with an increased risk for heart attack, stroke and sudden cardiac death. Growing evidence suggests that the higher your CRP level, the higher your risk of heart attack, even if you have no other indicators of heart disease. New studies have provided strong evidence that inflammation is a better predictor than cholesterol levels of your risk for heart disease.

Here's the dilemma doctors are currently faced with. CRP is simply a marker for CHD. There is no evidence available at this time that indicates lowering CRP levels with medication can actually reduce risk for CHD. Until there is sufficient evidence demonstrating the benefit of using medication to lower CRP levels, there is no real value in the test.

Homocysteine

As with CRP, there is no evidence at this time that indicates lowering homocysteine levels in the blood can actually reduce CHD risk. Until sufficient evidence becomes available, a test is of little value.

Lipoprotein-A

Lipoprotein-A is a type of blood fat. Your doctor may check your Lp(A) level if you or a family member has early-onset CAD. The treatment of elevated Lp(A) levels has been controversial. It is not yet known if lowering Lp(A) levels can actually reduce cardiovascular disease risk. For this reason, I see no benefit to this test at this time.

Electrocardiogram (ECG)

ECG is a painless test that measures the electrical activity of the heart. It can reveal several different heart problems. The test takes just a few minutes. You lie on a table with electrodes fastened to the skin of your chest, arms, and legs. Request one at age 35 to establish a baseline measure of heart function.

Exercise Stress Test

This test involves measuring ECG tracings before, during, and after stressing the heart by exercise. You will walk on a treadmill while connected to an ECG machine. This test is 60-70 percent accurate in showing blockages in blood flow in one or more of the three coronary arteries. Sometimes its readings may be falsely abnormal for people taking certain medications or who have certain medical problems not directly related to CHD.

Historically speaking, treadmill stress tests have failed to identify many future heart attack victims. This test had reportedly failed to identify the serious heart disease that former President Clinton underwent surgery for in 2005. Nonetheless, if you are experiencing symptoms of heart disease such as chest pain, shortness of breath or lightheadedness, you should speak to your doctor about this test. If your stress test is positive, your doctor will likely order an angiogram to help determine the extent of any blockages in blood vessels that supply the heart.

EBCT (Coronary Calcium Scan)

EBCT is a new and noninvasive but somewhat controversial test. By measuring the amount of calcium deposited in the plaques of coronary arteries, it can detect blockages of only 10-20 percent of an artery, which may not show up in other tests.

Three recent studies published in leading medical journals, including the *Journal of the American Medical Association*, found the scans to be of benefit in detecting heart attack risk. Dr. Scott Grundy, a researcher who drafted guidelines for the use of statin drugs for the National Cholesterol Education Program, believes the scans are as important as cholesterol tests in determining heart attack risk. Many groups are now recommending that men older than 45 and women older than 55 with traditional risk factors have the scan. The entire process takes about 15 minutes at a cost of roughly $400. The downside to this test is exposure to radiation, though minimal.

Cancer

Pap Examination for Cervical Cancer

No cancer screening test in medical history is as effective for early detection of cervical cancer as the Pap smear. Since the Pap examination was introduced, death rates from cervical cancer have dropped 70 percent in the U.S. Of women who do die of cervical cancer, 80 percent have not had a Pap examination in five years or more.

Every woman should have an annual Pap examination when she becomes sexually active or turns 18—whichever comes first. Regular Pap examinations should continue after menopause and after a hysterectomy (removal of the uterus). With early detection, cervical pre-cancer or cancer can be treated with a high probability of cure. The pelvic exam is added insurance; it can help detect signs of cancer in female organs other than the cervix.

Spiral CT Scan for Lung Cancer

The spiral CT scan is recommended for smokers or former smokers. This amazing technology can detect cancer when it's the size of a grain of rice. The scan takes an average of 20 seconds to perform and is generally not covered by insurance if for preventative purposes.

Colonoscopy for Colorectal Cancer

Colonoscopy allows a physician to look inside your entire large intestine, from the lowest part, the rectum, all the way up through the colon to the lower end of the small intestine. The procedure is used to look for early signs of cancer in the colon and rectum. It also allows the doctor to see abnormal growths, ulcers, inflamed tissue and bleeding.

For the procedure, you will lie on your left side on the examining table. You will probably be given pain medication and a mild sedative to keep you comfortable. The doctor will insert a long, flexible, lighted tube (colonoscope) into your rectum and slowly guide it into your colon. If anything abnormal is seen, like a polyp or inflamed tissue, it can be removed using tiny instruments passed through the scope and sent to a lab for testing. The exam takes approximately 30 to 60 minutes. Bleeding and puncture of the colon are possible complications of colonoscopy, though uncommon.

A newer test known as a virtual colonoscopy is now being offered. The problem remains that if something abnormal is detected on the virtual exam, you must still undergo a follow-up traditional exam to obtain a biopsy of the abnormal tissue.

PSA for Prostate Cancer

PSA (prostate-specific antigen) is a protein produced by the cells of the prostate gland. The PSA test measures the level of PSA in the blood. There is no specific normal or abnormal PSA level. However, the higher a man's PSA level, the more likely it is that cancer is present. If a man's PSA levels have been increasing or if a suspicious lump is detected during a digital rectal exam, additional tests such as a biopsy may be recommended to determine if there is cancer or another problem in the prostate.

Using the PSA test to screen men for prostate cancer is controversial because it is not yet known if the PSA test can actually save lives. Moreover, it is not clear if the benefits of PSA screening outweigh the risks of follow-up diagnostic tests and cancer treatments. For example, the PSA test may detect small cancers that would never become life threatening. The procedure used to diagnose prostate cancer (prostate biopsy) may cause side effects, including bleeding and infection. Prostate cancer treatment may cause incontinence (inability to control urine flow) and erectile dysfunction. For these reasons, it is important that the benefits and risks of diagnostic procedures and treatment be taken into account. A second opinion is always advised prior to undergoing any type of invasive treatment.

BRCA1 and BRCA2 for Breast and Ovarian Cancers

A woman's lifetime chance of developing breast and/or ovarian cancer is greatly increased if she inherits an altered BRCA1 or BRCA2 gene. Women with an inherited mutation in one of these genes have an increased risk of developing these cancers at a young age (before menopause), and often have multiple close family members with the disease.

These women may also have a greater chance of developing colon cancer. Men with an altered BRCA1 or BRCA2 gene also have an increased risk of breast cancer and possibly prostate cancer. A positive test result provides information only about a person's risk of developing cancer. It cannot tell whether cancer will actually develop—or when. Women with a high risk for breast cancer should speak to their doctor about this test. For others, it's probably of little to no benefit.

Mammography for Breast Cancer

The National Cancer Institute recommends that women begin receiving screening mammograms every one to two years at 40 years of age and every year once they reach 50. Many of the cancers that end up killing women were missed on X-ray mammography. Digital images can be enhanced by changing contrasts and magnified to view isolated areas. They also require less radiation than X-ray imaging and are easier to produce, store and transmit. Opt for a digital mammogram during your next screening exam.

Miscellaneous

Blood Glucose Test for Diabetes

The blood glucose test is ordered to measure the amount of glucose (sugar) in the blood. It is used to detect both high blood sugar (hyperglycemia) and low blood sugar (hypoglycemia) and to help diagnose diabetes. High levels of blood glucose most frequently indicate diabetes, but can also be caused by other diseases.

A blood glucose test is especially important if you are over age 45, at risk for diabetes or currently experiencing symptoms of diabetes. Early detection is the key to managing diabetes, as it can help minimize long-term complications.

Abdominal Ultrasound Screening for Abdominal Aortic Aneurysm (AAA)

The abdominal portion of the aorta is the large vessel that supplies blood to the abdomen, pelvis and legs. An aneurysm is a weakening and ballooning in the artery wall. A ruptured aorta is almost always fatal and in many instances, without symptoms. An abdominal ultrasound is a simple, painless and safe test that can detect aneurysms, and surgery can correct them, if necessary. This test is beneficial to those 65 or older, those with a family history of aneurysm, smokers, people with high blood pressure, or any type of CAD.

DEXA Scan (Bone Mineral Density Test) for Osteoporosis (Brittle Bones)

DEXA is most often used to diagnose osteoporosis, a condition that often affects women after menopause but may also be found in men. The DEXA test can also assess your risk for developing fractures and is effective in tracking the effects of treatment for osteoporosis and other conditions that cause bone loss.

The patient is placed on the back and asked to keep still while a scanner comes over the area to be tested. An X-ray machine under the table fires X-rays towards the scanner. The scan is painless and takes 10-15 minutes. If your bone density is found to be low, treatments are available to help prevent fractures before they occur. The test is highly recommended for women who are post-menopausal (especially tall and thin women), have a personal or maternal history of hip fracture, use medications that are known to cause bone loss, have an overactive thyroid condition, and who have X-ray evidence of osteoporosis.

Dilated Eye Exam to Prevent Blindness and Stroke

Diabetic retinopathy (DR) is the most common eye condition related to diabetes, and the most serious. DR is the most frequent cause of new blindness amongst Americans 20 to 74. Patients without diabetic retinopathy who are screened by retinal photography have a 95 percent probability of remaining free of sight-threatening retinopathy over the next 5 years. An eye exam could also help identify people at an increased risk for stroke. The circulation of the eyes and brain are essentially identical. Damage to the retina can indicate vascular abnormalities in the brain that put a person at higher risk for stroke. If retinopathy is present, you may want to speak to your doctor about ordering additional diagnostic tests that can help evaluate the blood supply to the brain.

In a Nutshell

Early detection and treatment are the keys to surviving many life-threatening illnesses and diseases, especially when it comes to heart disease and cancer. The longer a specific disease has to develop in your body, the more difficult it becomes to treat. As we age, our risk for specific illnesses and diseases becomes greater. Many times the onset of these diseases can go unnoticed or undetected during routine medical exams due to the absence of symptoms. Remember, heart disease may not exhibit any symptoms until there is up to a 90 percent blockage in a coronary artery.

Adhering to the schedule of tests above may someday help save your life and avoid a premature death. I recommend going through the list and checking off each of the tests you have already completed for your age bracket. Those that have not been completed should be discussed with your doctor, especially if you fall into a high-risk category for a specific disease. Many individuals are reluctant to undergo a specific test (e.g., colonoscopy) because it may seem uncomfortable. Keep in mind that the test for a specific disease is never as uncomfortable as the treatment for that disease (e.g., blood test for cholesterol vs. heart bypass surgery).

Chapter 9 Goals:

- ✓ Stay current on all preventative medical tests.
- ✓ Locate your specific category and check off all tests that have been completed.
- ✓ Make it a point to speak to your doctor about ordering the remaining tests.
- ✓ Always keep a record of all test results.

Appendix A

Are You Stressed Out?

The Social Readjustment Rating Scale is commonly used by many health care professionals to evaluate the role stress may play in a patient's health problems. This scale was originally designed to help predict the likelihood of a person getting a severe disease due to stress. A number of events that we may face in life have been rated numerically according to their potential to cause disease. A total of 200 or more points in one year indicates the likelihood of getting a severe disease. This scale should only be used as a rough predictor, as everyone reacts to stressful events differently.

THE SOCIAL READJUSTMENT RATING SCALE

RANK	LIFE EVENT	MEAN VALUE
1	Death of a spouse	100
2	Divorce	73
3	Marital separation	65
4	Jail term	63
5	Death of a close family member	63
6	Personal injury or illness	53
7	Marriage	50
8	Fired at work	47
9	Marital reconciliation	45
10	Retirement	45
11	Change in health of a family member	44
12	Pregnancy	40
13	Sexual difficulties	39

14	Gain of a new family member	39
15	Business adjustment	39
16	Change in financial state	38
17	Death of a close friend	37
18	Change of career	36
19	Change in number of arguments with spouse	35
20	Large mortgage	31
21	Foreclosure of mortgage or loan	30
22	Change in job responsibilities	29
23	Son or daughter leaving home	29
24	Trouble with in-laws	29
25	Outstanding personal achievement	28
26	Spouse begins or stops work	26
27	Begin or end school	26
28	Change in living conditions	25
29	Revision of personal habits	24
30	Trouble with boss	23
31	Change in work hours or conditions	20
32	Change in residence	20
33	Change in schools	20
34	Change in recreation	19
35	Change in church activities	19
36	Change in social activities	18
37	Small mortgage	17
38	Change in sleeping habits	16
39	Change in the number of family get-togethers	15
40	Change in eating habits	15
41	Vacationing	13
42	Christmas	12
43	Minor violations of the law	11

Total Score:

Stress-Prone Personality Test

If you answer yes to two or more of the following questions, you may have a stress-prone personality. Type A personalities are more likely to experience higher levels of stress than other people.

1. Do you try and do more than one thing at a time?
2. Do you rush through your meals?
3. Are you compulsive about punctuality?
4. Do you find it difficult to relax?
5. Do others tell you to take things slower?
6. Do you interrupt others frequently while they are talking?
7. Are you accident prone?
8. Do you get impatient or upset if something or someone delays you (traffic jams, appointments, etc.)?

Appendix B

The Lifestyle Diary—A Blueprint for Healthy Living

The following pages contain one blank and several sample Lifestyle Diaries. The Lifestyle Diary is intended to be used as a "blueprint" for healthy living. The sample diaries are to be used as guidelines, so study them carefully. I highly recommend printing out several copies of the blank diary and using them to track your daily lifestyle patterns. You can print out blank copies of the Lifestyle Diary from my website at www.LongevityMadeEasy.com.

MENU PLANNER

Beverages
Purified water
Spring water
Filtered water
Club soda
Seltzer water
Sparkling mineral water
Green tea *
V-8 (low-sodium variety only) *
Pomegranate juice *
Orange juice
Red wine (women 1 glass daily /
    men 1-2 glasses daily) *

*Note: Avoid all beverages
containing artificial sweeteners. Limit
consumption of beverages high in
sugar (10 grams or more per serving)*

Hot Cereals
Oatmeal (regular flavor only) *
Oat bran *
Unprocessed bran *

Cold Cereals
Cheerios *
Quaker Oat Bran *
Kashi Heart to Heart *
Kellogg's Complete Oat Bran Flakes *
Uncle Sam *
Safeway Select Organic Oat Bran Flakes *

*Note: Even cereals purchased from health
food markets can contain high amounts
of sugar and fat. Always read the product
label and search for cereals low in sugar
(< 10 grams per serving) and fat, and high
in fiber*

Vegetables
Spinach *
Broccoli *
Cauliflower
Tomato *
Garlic
Sweet potato
Brussels sprouts
Artichoke
Onion
Pepper
Celery
Asparagus
Mushrooms
Cucumbers
Green beans
Snap peas
Snow peas
Avocado
Red cabbage
Brussels sprouts
Squash
Bean sprouts
Radish
Swiss chard
Eggplant
Romaine lettuce
Kale
Endive

Fish, Meat and Other Proteins
Beef (free-range variety w/ all visible fat trimmed)
Chicken (free-range variety grilled and skinned w/ all visible fat trimmed)
Turkey
Venison
Salmon (wild variety only) *
Tilapia
Flounder
Trout
Sea Bass
Halibut
Mahi Mahi
Shellfish (limit consumption due to high cholesterol content)
Eggs (scrambled, hard-boiled, poached)

Note: Limit consumption of red meat to no more than once weekly

Nuts & Seeds
Walnuts *
Pecans *
Almonds *
Flaxseeds
Sunflower seeds
Peanut butter (natural varieties only)

Note: Raw and unsalted varieties

Beans
Black beans
Pinto beans
Kidney beans
Chick peas
Lentils
Garbanzo beans
Navy

Fruits
Blueberries *
Strawberries
Apples *
Cherries
Cranberries
Grapefruit
Orange
Pear
Bananas
Raspberries
Kiwifruit
Plum
Lemon and Lime

Dairy
Yogurt
Milk (skim, 1% or 2% varieties)
Cheese (in limited amounts)

*Note: Most people are under the false assumption that all yogurt is healthy. This
is not the case. Many yogurts contain high amounts of sugar, artificial colors
and flavors, and artificial sweeteners, making them far from healthy. Stick with
non-fat and low-fat plain varieties of yogurt. For flavor, try adding some fresh
blueberries, strawberries, peaches, bananas or nuts.*

Snacks
Baked tortilla chips w/ hummus or salsa
Celery or carrot sticks w/ peanut butter
Apple w/ peanut butter
Unbuttered popcorn
Unsalted pretzels
Sliced strawberries or blueberries w/ fat-free half and half
Frozen fruit (berries and cherries)
Dark chocolate (minimum of 70% cocoa)
Nuts (raw and unsalted)
Raw vegetables
Yogurt (non-fat or low-fat plain w/ fresh fruit)

Soups
All low-sodium, broth-based
varieties

*Note: Avoid cream-based
varieties of soup as they are
very high in fat and calories.*

*Denotes Daily Dozen Food Items

LONGEVITY DIARY

Day: _____   Give Yourself a Wellness Grade for Today: (A) (B) (C) (D) (F)

MEAL #1   Time: _____

_____
_____
_____
_____

SNACK #1   Time: _____

_____
_____

MEAL #2   Time: _____

_____
_____
_____

SNACK #2   Time: _____

_____
_____

MEAL #3   Time: _____

_____
_____
_____

SNACK #3   Time: _____

_____
_____

DAILY DOZEN FOODS*
- Tomato/Tomato Products
- Broccoli
- Spinach
- Whole Grains
- Fish (See Recommendations)
- Legumes
- Nuts
- Blueberries
- Apple
- Pomegranate Juice
- Green Tea
- Red Wine (See Recommendations)

SECONDARY FOODS
- Peanut Butter
- Yogurt
- Spices
- Avocado
- Sweet Potato
- Dark Chocolate/Cocoa

NUTRITIONAL SUPPLEMENTS
- Daily Multivitamin/Mineral
- Vitamin E (400 IUs)
- Vitamin C (500 mg)
- Selenium (200 mcg)
- Fish Oil/Flax Seed Oil (1-2 grams)
- Garlic Extract (600 mg twice daily)
- Green Tree Extract (300-400 mg)
- B-Complex Vitamin (as directed)
- Calcium Citrate (800-1200 mg)
- Fiber (Optional: 25-35 grams daily)
- Co-Q10 (Optional: 100-150 mg)
- Aspirin (Physician Supervised)

WATER
- 8 Eight Ounce Glasses or More Daily

SLEEP QUALITY**
- Hours: 1·2·3·4·5·6·7·8·9·10·11·12
- Quality: Poor·Fair·Good·Excellent

PHYSICAL ACTIVITY
- Aerobic Activity
  Type:
  Duration:
- Weight Training
- Yoga
- Pilates
- Other:

RELAXATION TECHNIQUES
- Deep Breathing
- Progressive Relaxation
- T'ai Chi
- Yoga
- Meditation
- Laughter

SOCIAL NETWORKS***
- Socialized with Friends Today

INTELLECTUAL ACTIVITY
- Reading, Puzzles, Problem Solving

TODAY I FEEL...
- Happy
- Sad
- Depressed
- Lonely
- Angry
- Frustrated
- Hopeless
- Anxious

PHYSICAL ASSESSMENT****
- Weight (lbs):
- Bodyfat:
- BMI:
- Waist Circumference:
- Improvement: ○ Yes   ○ No

DAILY STRESS METER

Very Low   Moderate   Very High

*   Consume as many foods as possible each day from this group.
** 7-8 hours of sleep per night is recommended.
*** Socialized with people other than family members.
****Physical assesment should be performed bi-weekly to evaluate for improvement.

LONGEVITY DIARY

Day: Monday   Give Yourself a Wellness Grade for Today: (A) (B) (C) (D) (F)

MEAL #1   Time: 8:50 a.m.

Instant Oatmeal with Blueberries and Oat Bran (2 tbsp)

Scrambled Eggs (2 whites/2 whole eggs w/ non-stick cooking spray)

Pomegranate Juice (8 oz)

Coffee w/ half and half (no sugar)

SNACK #1   Time: 11:00 a.m.

Apple w/natural peanut butter (2 tbsp)

MEAL #2   Time: 1:20 p.m.

Garden salad w/baby spinach, tomatoes, broccoli, cauliflower, avocado and goat cheese

Sliced grilled free-range chicken breast

Olive oil (2 tbsp) and balsamic vinegar mix for dressing

Green tea with lemon (2 cups)

SNACK #2   Time: 3:30 p.m.

Protein shake (whey) with non-fat milk and cinnamon

Walnuts (about a handful)

MEAL #3   Time: 6:00 p.m.

Wild salmon w/ lemon and herbs (baked)

Broccoli (steamed) with lemon and olive oil

Garden salad w/ baby spinach, cabbage, tomatoes, onions and cucumbers

Olive Oil (2 tbsp) and balsamic vinegar mix for dressing

Red Wine (1 glass)

SNACK #3   Time: 8:20 p.m.

Green tea (2 cups)

Dark Chocolate (70% cocoa)

DAILY DOZEN FOODS*
- ☑ Tomato/Tomato Products
- ☑ Broccoli
- ☑ Spinach
- ☑ Whole Grains
- ☑ Fish (See Recommendations)
- ☑ Legumes
- ☑ Nuts
- ☑ Blueberries
- ☑ Apple
- ☑ Pomegranate Juice
- ☑ Green Tea
- ☑ Red Wine (See Recommendations)

SECONDARY FOODS
- ☑ Peanut Butter
- ☑ Yogurt
- ☐ Spices
- ☑ Avocado
- ☑ Sweet Potato
- ☑ Dark Chocolate/Cocoa

NUTRITIONAL SUPPLEMENTS
- ☑ Daily Multivitamin/Mineral
- ☑ Vitamin E (400 IUs)
- ☑ Vitamin C (500 mg)
- ☑ Selenium (200 mcg)
- ☑ Fish Oil/Flax Seed Oil (1-2 grams)
- ☑ Garlic Extract (600 mg twice daily)
- ☑ Green Tea Extract (300-400 mg)
- ☑ B-Complex Vitamin (as directed)
- ☑ Calcium Citrate (800-1200 mg)
- ☐ Fiber (Optional: 25-35 grams daily)
- ☐ Co-Q10 (Optional: 100-150 mg)
- ☐ Aspirin (Physician Supervised)

WATER
- ☑ 8 Eight Ounce Glasses or More Daily

SLEEP QUALITY**
- ☑ Hours: 1•2•3•4•5•6•7•8•9•10•11•12
- ☑ Quality: Poor•Fair•Good•Excellent

PHYSICAL ACTIVITY
- ☑ Aerobic Activity
  Type: Treadmill
  Duration: 45 minutes
- ☑ Weight Training
- ☐ Yoga
- ☐ Pilates
- ☐ Other:

RELAXATION TECHNIQUES
- ☑ Deep Breathing
- ☐ Progressive Relaxation
- ☐ Tai Chi
- ☐ Yoga
- ☐ Meditation
- ☑ Laughter

SOCIAL NETWORKS***
- ☑ Socialized with Friends Today

INTELLECTUAL ACTIVITY
- ☑ Reading, Puzzles, Problem Solving

TODAY I FEEL...
- ☑ Happy   ☐ Angry
- ☐ Sad   ☐ Frustrated
- ☐ Depressed   ☐ Hopeless
- ☐ Lonely   ☐ Anxious

PHYSICAL ASSESSMENT****
- ☑ Weight (lbs): 205
- ☑ Bodyfat: 19%
- ☑ BMI: 2.5
- ☑ Waist Circumference: 32 inches
- ☑ Improvement: ☑ Yes   ☐ No

DAILY STRESS METER

Very Low   Moderate   Very High

(X marked near Moderate/Very Low)

---

*   Consume as many foods as possible each day from the group.

**   7-8 hours of sleep per night is recommended.

***   Socialized with people other than family members.

****   Physical assessment should be performed bi-weekly to evaluate for improvement.

LONGEVITY DIARY

Day: Tuesday **Give Yourself a Wellness Grade for Today:** (A) (B) (C) (D) (F)

MEAL #1 Time: 8:40 a.m.
Instant Oatmeal with Blueberries and Oat Bran (2 tbsp)
Protein shake (whey) with low-fat milk and cinnamon
Pomegranate juice (8 oz)
Coffee with half and half (no sugar)

SNACK #1 Time: 10:55 a.m.
Yogurt (non-fat plain) with fresh strawberries

MEAL #2 Time: 1:15 p.m.
Garden salad w/baby spinach, tomatoes, broccoli, onions, chick peas, walnuts and walnuts
Olive oil (2 tbsp) and balsamic vinegar for dressing
Italian wedding soup (bowl)
Green tea with lemon (2 cups)

SNACK #2 Time: 3:10 p.m.
Protein Shake (low-sugar ready-to-drink variety)
Walnuts (handful)

MEAL #3 Time: 5:45 p.m.
Free-range chicken with lemon, garlic and herbs (baked)
Asparagus (steamed) with lemon, olive oil and light parmesan cheese
Sweet potato with low-fat sour cream (1 tbsp)
Red wine (2 glasses)
Coffee with half and half (no sugar)

SNACK #3 Time: 7:30 p.m.
Apple with peanut butter (1 tbsp)

SLEEP QUALITY**
☑ Hours: 1•2•3•4•5•6•7•8•9•10•11•12
☑ Quality: Poor•Fair•Good•Excellent

PHYSICAL ACTIVITY
☑ Aerobic Activity
  Type: Elliptical trainer
  Duration: 45 minutes
○ Weight Training
○ Yoga
○ Pilates
○ Other:

RELAXATION TECHNIQUES
○ Deep Breathing
○ Progressive Relaxation
○ Tai Chi
○ Yoga
○ Meditation
☑ Laughter

SOCIAL NETWORKS***
☑ Socialized with Friends Today

INTELLECTUAL ACTIVITY
☑ Reading, Puzzles, Problem Solving

TODAY I FEEL...
○ Happy   ○ Angry
○ Sad   ○ Frustrated
○ Depressed ○ Hopeless
○ Lonely   ☑ Anxious

PHYSICAL ASSESSMENT****
☑ Weight (lbs): 205
☑ Bodyfat: 8%
☑ BMI: 25
☑ Waist Circumference: 32 inches
☑ Improvement: ☑Yes ○No

DAILY DOZEN FOODS*
☑ Tomato/Tomato Products
☑ Broccoli
☑ Spinach
☑ Whole Grains
☑ Fish (See Recommendations)
☑ Legumes
☑ Nuts
☑ Blueberries
☑ Apple
☑ Pomegranate Juice
☑ Green Tea
☑ Red Wine (See Recommendations)

SECONDARY FOODS
☑ Peanut Butter
☑ Yogurt
☑ Spices
☑ Avocado
☑ Sweet Potato
☑ Dark Chocolate/Cocoa

NUTRITIONAL SUPPLEMENTS
☑ Daily Multivitamin/Mineral
☑ Vitamin E (400 IUs)
☑ Vitamin C (500 mg)
☑ Selenium (200 mcg)
☑ Fish Oil/Flax Seed Oil (1-2 grams)
☑ Garlic Extract (600 mg twice daily)
☑ Green Tea Extract (300-400 mg)
☑ B-Complex Vitamin (as directed)
☑ Calcium Citrate (800-1200 mg)
☑ Fiber (Optional: 25-35 grams daily)
○ Co-Q10 (Optional: 100-150 mg)
○ Aspirin (Physician Supervised)

WATER
☑ 8 Eight Ounce Glasses or More Daily

DAILY STRESS METER

Very Low   Moderate   Very High

---

*   Consume as many foods as possible each day from this group.
**   7-8 hours of sleep per night is recommended.
***   Socialized with people other than family members.
**** Physical assessment should be performed bi-weekly to evaluate for improvement.

LONGEVITY DIARY

Day: Tuesday **Give Yourself a Wellness Grade for Today:** Ⓐ Ⓑ Ⓒ Ⓓ Ⓕ

MEAL #1 **Time:** 8:45 a.m.

Whole grain low-sugar cereal with fresh blueberries and low-fat milk

Protein shake (50/50 soy and whey) with non-fat milk and cinnamon

Pomegranate juice (8 ounces)

Coffee with half and half (no sugar)

SNACK #1 **Time:** 10:30 a.m.

Apple w/ peanut butter

Green tea w/ lemon and honey (2 cups - 1 tsp of honey per cup)

MEAL #2 **Time:** 12:0 p.m.

Garden salad w/baby spinach, tomatoes, broccoli, cauliflower, avocado and chick peas

Olive oil (2 tbsp) and balsamic vinegar mix for dressing

Black bean soup (bowl)

Coffee with half and half (no sugar)

SNACK #2 **Time:** 3:30 p.m.

Protein shake (whey) with non-fat milk and cinnamon

Walnuts (about a handful)

MEAL #3 **Time:** 5:50 p.m.

Vegetarian chili w/beans (no meat added - added black beans and onions)

Whole grain bread (2 slices)

Red wine (2 glasses)

Homemade cocoa with soy milk and 1-2 tsp of sugar

SNACK #3 **Time:** 7:50 p.m.

Yogurt (low-fat, plain) with frozen blueberries

DAILY DOZEN FOODS*
- ☑ Tomato/Tomato Products
- ☑ Broccoli
- ☑ Spinach
- ☑ Whole Grains
- ☐ Fish (See Recommendations)
- ☑ Legumes
- ☑ Nuts
- ☑ Blueberries
- ☑ Apple
- ☑ Pomegranate Juice
- ☑ Green Tea
- ☑ Red Wine (See Recommendations)

SECONDARY FOODS
- ☑ Peanut Butter
- ☑ Yogurt
- ☐ Spices
- ☑ Avocado
- ☐ Sweet Potato
- ☑ Dark Chocolate/Cocoa

NUTRITIONAL SUPPLEMENTS
- ☑ Daily Multivitamin/Mineral
- ☑ Vitamin E (400 IUs)
- ☑ Vitamin C (500 mg)
- ☑ Selenium (200 mcg)
- ☑ Fish Oil/Flax Seed Oil (1-2 grams)
- ☑ Garlic Extract (600 mg twice daily)
- ☑ Green Tea Extract (300-400 mg)
- ☑ B-Complex Vitamin (as directed)
- ☑ Calcium Citrate (800-1200 mg)
- ☐ Fiber (Optional: 25-35 grams daily)
- ☐ Co-Q10 (Optional: 100-150 mcg)
- ☐ Aspirin (Physician Supervised)

WATER
- ☑ 8 Eight Ounce Glasses or More Daily

SLEEP QUALITY**
- ☑ Hours: 1•2•3•4•5•6•7•8•9•10•11•12
- ☑ Quality: Poor-Fair-Good-Excellent

PHYSICAL ACTIVITY
- ☑ Aerobic Activity
  Type: Spinning Class
  Duration: 6-0 minutes
- ☑ Weight Training
- ☐ Yoga
- ☐ Pilates
- ☐ Other:

RELAXATION TECHNIQUES
- ☐ Deep Breathing
- ☐ Progressive Relaxation
- ☐ Tai Chi
- ☐ Yoga
- ☐ Meditation
- ☐ Laughter

SOCIAL NETWORKS***
- ☑ Socialized with Friends Today

INTELLECTUAL ACTIVITY
- ☑ Reading, Puzzles, Problem Solving

TODAY I FEEL...
- ☐ Happy
- ☐ Sad
- ☐ Lonely
- ☐ Angry
- ☑ Frustrated
- ☐ Depressed
- ☐ Hopeless
- ☐ Anxious

PHYSICAL ASSESSMENT****
- Weight (lbs):
- Bodyfat:
- BMI:
- Waist Circumference:
- Improvement: ☐ Yes ☐ No

DAILY STRESS METER

Very Low　　Moderate　　Very High

X

* Consume as many foods as possible each day from this group.
** 7-8 hours of sleep per night is recommended.
*** Socialized with people other than family members.
**** Physical assessment should be performed weekly to evaluate for improvement.

LONGEVITY DIARY

Day: Thursday **Give Yourself a Wellness Grade for Today:** (A) (B) (C) (D) (F)

MEAL #1   **Time:** 9:10 a.m.

Eggs (4 hard boiled)

Whole grain toast (w/ Smart Balance spread)

Apple

V-8 juice (low sodium)

Coffee with half and half (no sugar)

SNACK #1   **Time:** 11:20 a.m.

Meal-replacement bar (high-protein, low carbohydrate)

Green tea with lemon and honey (1 tsp)

MEAL #2   **Time:** 1:20 p.m.

Garden salad w/baby spinach, cabbage, tomatoes, broccoli, cauliflower, onion and avocado

Olive oil (2 tbsp) and balsamic vinegar mix for dressing

Pasta fazool soup (Italian pasta and bean soup-tuna)

Pomegranate juice

SNACK #2   **Time:** 3:30 p.m.

Protein shake (whey) with soy milk and cinnamon

Walnuts (about a handful)

MEAL #3   **Time:** 5:45 p.m.

Grilled free-range chicken breast with lemon, garlic and herbs

Garden salad w/ baby spinach, tomatoes, onions, chick peas, black beans and cucumber

Olive oil (2 tbsp) and balsamic vinegar mix for dressing

Red wine (2 glasses)

Green tea with lemon and honey (1 tsp)

SNACK #3   **Time:** 7:30 p.m.

Baked tortilla chips with hummus

Dark chocolate bar (4 oz.)

DAILY DOZEN FOODS*

- ☑ Tomato/Tomato Products
- ☑ Broccoli
- ☑ Spinach
- ☑ Whole Grains
- ☐ Fish (See Recommendations)
- ☑ Legumes
- ☑ Nuts
- ☑ Blueberries
- ☑ Apple
- ☑ Pomegranate Juice
- ☑ Green Tea
- ☑ Red Wine (See Recommendations)

SECONDARY FOODS

- ☐ Peanut Butter
- ☐ Yogurt
- ☐ Spices
- ☑ Avocado
- ☐ Sweet Potato
- ☑ Dark Chocolate/Cocoa

NUTRITIONAL SUPPLEMENTS

- ☑ Daily Multivitamin/Mineral
- ☑ Vitamin E (400 IUs)
- ☑ Vitamin C (500 mg)
- ☑ Selenium (200 mcg)
- ☑ Fish Oil/Flax Seed Oil (1-2 grams)
- ☑ Garlic Extract (600 mg twice daily)
- ☑ Green Tea Extract (300-400 mg)
- ☑ B-Complex Vitamin (as directed)
- ☑ Calcium Citrate (800-1200 mg)
- ☐ Fiber (Optional: 25-35 grams daily)
- ☐ Co-Q10 (Optional: 100-150 mg)
- ☐ Aspirin (Physician Supervised)

WATER

☑ 8 Eight Ounce Glasses or More Daily

SLEEP QUALITY**

- ☑ Hours: 1•2•3•4•5•6•7•8•9•10•11•12
- ☑ Quality: Poor•Fair•Good•Excellent

PHYSICAL ACTIVITY

- ☑ Aerobic Activity
  Type: Treadmill
  Duration: 60 minutes
- ☐ Weight Training
- ☐ Yoga
- ☐ Pilates
- ☐ Other:

RELAXATION TECHNIQUES

- ☑ Deep Breathing
- ☐ Progressive Relaxation
- ☐ Tai Chi
- ☐ Yoga
- ☑ Meditation
- ☑ Laughter

SOCIAL NETWORKS***

☑ Socialized with Friends Today

INTELLECTUAL ACTIVITY

☑ Reading, Puzzles, Problem Solving

TODAY I FEEL...

- ☑ Happy
- ☐ Sad
- ☐ Depressed
- ☐ Lonely
- ☐ Angry
- ☐ Frustrated
- ☐ Hopeless
- ☐ Anxious

PHYSICAL ASSESSMENT****

- ☐ Weight (lbs):
- ☐ Bodyfat:
- ☐ BMI:
- ☐ Waist Circumference:
- ☐ Improvement: ☐ Yes ☐ No

DAILY STRESS METER

Very Low   Moderate   Very High

---

* Consume as many foods as possible each day from this group.

** 7-8 hours of sleep per night is recommended.

*** Socialized with people other than family members.

**** Physical assessment should be performed bi-weekly to evaluate to improvement.

LONGEVITY DIARY

Day: Friday   Give Yourself a Wellness Grade for Today: (A) (B) (C) (D) (F)

MEAL #1   Time: 8:45 a.m.
Cold whole grain low-sugar cereal with skim milk and fresh blueberries added
4 scrambled egg whites
Pomegranate juice (8 oz)
Coffee w/ half and half (no sugar)

SNACK #1   Time: 10:30 a.m.
Protein shake (whey) with non-fat milk and cinnamon

MEAL #2   Time: 12:40 p.m.
Garden salad w/baby spinach, cabbage, tomatoes, broccoli, cauliflower, chick peas, onions and goat cheese
Italian wedding soup (cup)
Olive oil (2 tbsp) and balsamic vinegar for dressing
Green tea (2 cups w/ lemon)

SNACK #2   Time: 2:50 p.m.
Walnuts (about 2 handfuls)
Apple

MEAL #3   Time: 5:25 p.m.
Tilapia (baked) w/ lemon and herbs
Steamed broccoli w/ lemon, garlic and olive oil
Sweet potato w/ low-fat sour cream
Red wine (2 glasses)
Coffee w/ half and half (no sugar)

SNACK #3   Time: 7:30 p.m.
Dark chocolate bar (4 oz)
Green tea (2 cups with lemon)

DAILY DOZEN FOODS*
- ☑ Tomato/Tomato Products
- ☑ Broccoli
- ☑ Spinach
- ☑ Whole Grains
- ☑ Fish (See Recommendations)
- ☑ Legumes
- ☑ Nuts
- ☑ Blueberries
- ☑ Apple
- ☑ Pomegranate Juice
- ☑ Green Tea
- ☑ Red Wine (See Recommendations)

SECONDARY FOODS
- ☐ Peanut Butter
- ☐ Yogurt
- ☐ Spices
- ☐ Avocado
- ☑ Sweet Potato
- ☑ Dark Chocolate/Cocoa

NUTRITIONAL SUPPLEMENTS
- ☑ Daily Multivitamin/Mineral
- ☑ Vitamin E (400 IUs)
- ☑ Vitamin C (500 mg)
- ☑ Selenium (200 mcg)
- ☑ Fish Oil/Flax Seed Oil (1-2 grams)
- ☑ Garlic Extract (600 mg twice daily)
- ☑ Green Tea Extract (300-400 mg)
- ☑ B-Complex Vitamin (as directed)
- ☑ Calcium Citrate (800-1200 mg)
- ☑ Fiber (Optional: 25-35 grams daily)
- ☐ Co-Q10 (Optional: 100-150 mg)
- ☐ Aspirin (Physician Supervised)

WATER
- ☑ 8 Eight Ounce Glasses or More Daily

SLEEP QUALITY**
- ☑ Hours: 1•2•3•4•5•6•7•8•9•10•11•12
- ☑ Quality: Poor•Fair•Good•Excellent

PHYSICAL ACTIVITY
- ☑ Aerobic Activity
  Type: Biking
  Duration: 45 minutes
- ☑ Weight Training
- ☐ Yoga
- ☐ Pilates
- ☐ Other:

RELAXATION TECHNIQUES
- ☑ Deep Breathing
- ☐ Progressive Relaxation
- ☐ Tai Chi
- ☐ Yoga
- ☐ Meditation
- ☑ Laughter

SOCIAL NETWORKS***
- ☑ Socialized with Friends Today

INTELLECTUAL ACTIVITY
- ☑ Reading, Puzzles, Problem Solving

TODAY I FEEL
- ☑ Happy
- ☐ Sad
- ☐ Depressed
- ☐ Lonely
- ☐ Angry
- ☐ Frustrated
- ☐ Hopeless
- ☐ Anxious

PHYSICAL ASSESSMENT****
- ☐ Weight (lbs):
- ☐ Body-fat:
- ☐ BMI:
- ☐ Waist Circumference:
- ☐ Improvement: ☐ Yes   ☐ No

DAILY STRESS METER

Very Low	Moderate	Very High

X

* Consume as many foods as possible each day from this group.
** 7-8 hours of sleep per night is recommended.
*** Socialized with people other than family members.
**** Physical assement should be performed bi-weekly to evaluate for improvement.

LONGEVITY DIARY

Day: Saturday Give Yourself a Wellness Grade for Today: (A) (B) (C) (D) (F)

MEAL #1   Time: 6:30 a.m.

Omelet w/ spinach, tomato and feta cheese (non-stick cooking spray)

Whole grain toast (2 slices w/ Smart Balance spread)

Apple

Pomegranate juice

Coffee w/ 2 tbsp half and half (no sugar)

SNACK #1   Time: 10:45 a.m.

Protein shake (whey) with soy milk and cinnamon

_____

_____

MEAL #2   Time: 1:20 p.m.

Pizza (3 slices)

Iced tea (sweetened with 2 packets of sugar)

_____

SNACK #2   Time: 2:50 p.m.

Tomato and mozzarella cheese (sliced) w/ olive oil, balsamic vinegar and fresh basil

Walnuts (handful)

_____

MEAL #3   Time: 5:20 p.m.

Filet Mignon (grilled 8 oz.)

Garden salad w/ baby spinach, tomato, walnuts and goat cheese (olive oil and vinegar)

Asparagus (grilled and topped with olive oil and lemon juice)

Red wine (2 glasses)

Coffee with half and half (no sugar)

SNACK #3   Time: 8:40 p.m.

Dark chocolate bar (4 oz.)

Green tea (2 cups)

_____

DAILY DOZEN FOODS*
- ☑ Tomato/Tomato Products
- ☐ Broccoli
- ☐ Spinach
- ☑ Whole Grains
- ☑ Fish (See Recommendations)
- ☐ Legumes
- ☑ Nuts
- ☐ Blueberries
- ☑ Apple
- ☑ Pomegranate Juice
- ☑ Green Tea
- ☑ Red Wine (See Recommendations)

SECONDARY FOODS
- ☐ Peanut Butter
- ☐ Yogurt
- ☐ Spices
- ☐ Avocado
- ☐ Sweet Potato
- ☑ Dark Chocolate/Cocoa

NUTRITIONAL SUPPLEMENTS
- ☑ Daily Multivitamin/Mineral
- ☑ Vitamin E (400 IUs)
- ☑ Vitamin C (500 mg)
- ☑ Selenium (200 mcg)
- ☑ Fish Oil/Flax Seed Oil (1-2 grams)
- ☑ Garlic Extract (600 mg twice daily)
- ☑ Green Tea Extract (300-400 mg)
- ☑ B-Complex Vitamin (as directed)
- ☑ Calcium Citrate (800-1200 mg)
- ☐ Fiber (Optional: 25-35 grams daily)
- ☐ Co-Q10 (Optional: 100-150 mg)
- ☐ Aspirin (Physician Supervised)

WATER
- ☑ 8 Eight Ounce Glasses or More Daily

SLEEP QUALITY**
- ☑ Hours: 1•2•3•4•5•6•7•8•9•10•11•12
- ☑ Quality: Poor•Fair•Good•Excellent

PHYSICAL ACTIVITY
- ☑ Aerobic Activity
  Type: Spinning Class
  Duration: 60 minutes
- ☑ Weight Training
- ☐ Yoga
- ☐ Pilates
- ☐ Other:

RELAXATION TECHNIQUES
- ☐ Deep Breathing
- ☐ Progressive Relaxation
- ☐ Tai Chi
- ☐ Yoga
- ☐ Meditation
- ☐ Laughter

SOCIAL NETWORKS***
- ☑ Socialized with Friends Today

INTELLECTUAL ACTIVITY
- ☐ Reading, Puzzles, Problem Solving

TODAY I FEEL...
- ☑ Happy
- ☐ Sad
- ☐ Depressed
- ☐ Lonely
- ☐ Angry
- ☐ Frustrated
- ☐ Hopeless
- ☐ Anxious

PHYSICAL ASSESSMENT****
- ☐ Weight (lbs):
- ☐ Body Fat:
- ☐ BMI:
- ☐ Waist Circumference:
- ☐ Improvement: ☐ Yes   ☐ No

DAILY STRESS METER

Very Low   Moderate   Very High

*   Consume as many foods as possible each day from this group.
**   7-8 hours of sleep per night is recommended.
*** Socialized with people other than family members.
**** Physical assessment should be performed bi-weekly to evaluate for improvement.

978-0-595-41184-9
0-595-41184-3